The Vulva

A Practi

S

The Vulva

A Practical Handbook for Clinicians

Second edition

Gayle Fischer
The University of Sydney, Australia

Jennifer Bradford
The University of Western Sydney, Australia

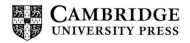

CAMBRIDGE
UNIVERSITY PRESS

University Printing House, Cambridge CB2 8BS, United Kingdom

Cambridge University Press is part of the University of Cambridge.

It furthers the University's mission by disseminating knowledge in the pursuit of education, learning and research at the highest international levels of excellence.

www.cambridge.org
Information on this title: www.cambridge.org/9781316508954

First published 2010 by Family Planning NSW
Second Edition by Cambridge University Press 2016
Reprinted 2016

Printed in the United Kingdom by Clays, St Ives plc

A catalogue record for this publication is available from the British Library

Library of Congress Cataloguing in Publication data
Names: Fischer, Gayle, 1953– author. | Bradford, Jennifer, 1960– author.
Title: The vulva : a practical handbook for clinicians / Gayle Fischer, Jennifer Bradford.
Description: Second edition. | Cambridge, United Kingdom ; New York : Cambridge University Press, 2016. | Includes bibliographical references and index.
Identifiers: LCCN 2016041185 | ISBN 9781316508954 (paperback : alk. paper)
Subjects: | MESH: Vulvar Diseases
Classification: LCC RG261 | NLM WP 200 | DDC 618.1/6 – dc23
LC record available at https://lccn.loc.gov/2016041185

ISBN 978-1-316-50895-4 Paperback

....

Every effort has been made in preparing this book to provide accurate and up-to-date information which is in accord with accepted standards and practice at the time of publication. Although case histories are drawn from actual cases, every effort has been made to disguise the identities of the individuals involved. Nevertheless, the authors, editors and publishers can make no warranties that the information contained herein is totally free from error, not least because clinical standards are constantly changing through research and regulation. The authors, editors and publishers therefore disclaim all liability for direct or consequential damages resulting from the use of material contained in this book. Readers are strongly advised to pay careful attention to information provided by the manufacturer of any drugs or equipment that they plan to use.

Contents

Foreword

This is the best comprehensive – yet concise – book on the recognition and management of vulvar diseases that I know: an excellent choice for gynaecologists, dermatologists and family practitioners. It is a practical text for the management of conditions that can at times be very complex and challenging.

Vulvar diseases are not a priority in the education of physicians and caregivers for women nor in any of the 'women's health initiatives'. These conditions are generally ignored in medical education at all levels. Women themselves generally have no genital education because they and their caregivers are educated under the prevailing cultural taboos. The result is that vulvar teaching is usually overlooked, so vulvar diseases are perceived as difficult to diagnose and treat.

This book is succinct, well organised and covers the basic aspects of the vulva with excellent diagrams. It is written in a simple format using point form that is easy to follow. Each chapter covers the clinical presentation, misconceptions and common questions for each condition. Each condition is addressed in a concise and helpful manner. Full-colour clinical photographs and illustrations demonstrate the clinical appearance of a wide spectrum of vulvar dermatoses and lesions. Excellent lists simplify management.

Co-written by a dermatologist and gynaecologist – both experienced clinicians and researchers specialising in vulvar conditions – the handbook provides a unique visual and written guide to the causes, diagnosis, treatment and management of both acute and chronic vulvar conditions. With its unique and practical 'how-to' approach, this comprehensive handbook is a must-have for health professionals learning to care for the most avoided and under-taught area in women's health.

Lynette J. Margesson MD FRCPC
Assistant Professor of Obstetrics & Gynecology and Surgery (Dermatology)
Geisel School of Medicine at Dartmouth, Hanover, NH, USA

Preface

The first edition of this book appeared in 2010, at a time when there was very little published evidence on vulval disease. Happily, the situation has improved, and the entire text has been amended to reflect this. Further reading lists are included at the end of the chapters. In the last 5 years, the authors themselves have completed important research on genital candidiasis, lichen planus, lichen sclerosus and persistent vaginitis. They have included a précis of this information, as well as relevant research from other centres.

Without accurate diagnosis, there can be no effective treatment. Even today, vulval problems are too often ignored or mismanaged. Our aim is to demystify vulval disease and explain how accurate diagnosis and effective treatment is not only possible but within the reach of clinicians everywhere.

Glossary

Acanthosis nigricans – a velvety eruption, sometimes with wart-like growths, accompanied by hyperpigmentation in the skin of the armpits, neck, anogenital area and groin

Alopecia areata – an autoimmune condition that causes hair loss with round bald patches, which can evolve to complete baldness

Amoebiasis – a tropical infection with *Entamoeba histolytica*, most commonly causing gastroenteritis

Angiokeratoma – harmless raised, purple lesions composed of blood vessels with a hyperkeratotic surface, often found on the labia majora

Apareunia – inability to perform coitus because of a physical or psychological sexual dysfunction

Aphthae – small, shallow, painful ulcers that usually affect the oral mucosa but less commonly affect the vulva

Atopy – a common genetic condition characterised by asthma, hay fever and dermatitis, as well as, in some patients, exaggerated IgE responses

Autoimmune thyroiditis – an inflammatory disease of the thyroid associated with high levels of thyroid autoantibodies

Bleb – a blister filled with fluid (see also Vesicle)

Campbell de Morgan spots – red papules on the skin containing a proliferation of blood vessels very commonly found in middle-aged people

Candidiasis – fungal infection caused by *Candida* species, most often *C. albicans*

Cellulitis – a bacterial skin infection characterised by spreading painful erythema, most often due to group A *Streptococcus*

Chancroid – sexually transmissible tropical infection caused by *Haemophilus ducreyi* and characterised by genital ulcers

Comedones – also known as blackheads: papules with a dark centre caused by a build-up of sebaceous material in hair follicles

Crohn's disease – an inflammatory disease that may affect any part of the gastrointestinal tract from mouth to anus, which causes a wide variety of symptoms

Cytokines – immunoregulatory chemicals

Dermoscopy – a technique for examining skin lesions using a hand-held magnifying device

Desquamation – shedding of the outer layers of the skin

Desquamative inflammatory vulvovaginitis – an uncommon chronic non-infective vulvovaginitis characterised by an introital and vaginal rash, soreness, dyspareunia and discharge

Dowling–Degos disease – a rare disease causing reticulated hyperpigmentation of the vulval and axillary skin

Dyspareunia – painful sexual intercourse

Erythema – redness of the skin

Folliculitis – inflammation or infection of one or more hair follicles characterised by a pustular eruption

Fomite – any inanimate object or substance capable of carrying infectious organisms

Fourchette – a small fold of membrane connecting the labia minora in the posterior part of the vulva

Fox–Fordyce disease – a rare skin disorder characterised by the development of itchy bumps around the hair follicles of the underarm area, pubic region, and/or around the nipples

Hamartoma – a neoplasm resulting from overgrowth of normal tissue

Hidradenitis suppurativa – a severe, chronic recurrent condition of the apocrine sweat glands characterised by nodules, pustules and sinuses

Hyperalgesia – pain or discomfort from light touch, intolerance of tight clothes

Inguinal – pertaining to the groin

Intertriginous – where two skin areas touch or rub together

Koebner phenomenon – refers to skin lesions appearing in areas of chronic trauma

Leishmaniasis – a skin disease characterised by ulcers and nodules caused by protozoan parasites of the genus *Leishmania* transmitted by sandfly bite

Lichenification – thickening of the surface of the skin caused by scratching

Lymphogranuloma venereum – a sexually transmissible disease caused by *Chlamydia trachomatis* causing genital abscesses and ulcers

Maceration – softening and whitening of skin due to chronic wetness

Macule – a change in skin colour without elevation or depression

Marsupialisation – cutting off the top of a cyst and suturing the cyst edges of the skin

Molluscum contagiosum – a viral skin disease characterised by small umbilicated papules

Morphoea – a condition in which there are areas of skin fibrosis similar to a scar

Mucosal petechiae – red–purple lesions of the skin or mucosa due extravasation of blood from capillaries

Naevi – birthmarks or coloured skin markings

Neurofibromatosis – a genetic disease in which patients develop multiple soft tumours (neurofibromas) under the skin and throughout the nervous system associated with pigmented skin lesions

Non-sexual acute genital ulceration (NSAGU) – aphthous ulceration of the vulva (see Aphthae)

Papilloma – a benign pedunculated tumour

Papillomatous – raised and rough, similar to a wart

Papules – firm raised lesions on the skin

Pedunculated – growing or attaching to a peduncle or stalk

Pernicious anaemia – anaemia due to vitamin B12 deficiency

Pruritus – itch

Punctum – the opening of a sebaceous cyst

Rugose – wrinkled or ridged

Sebaceous adenitis – recurrent inflammation of the sebaceous glands of the labia minora

Sebaceous hyperplasia – a common harmless enlargement of the skin oil glands, which features skin-coloured to yellow-white elevations of the skin

Seborrhoeic keratoses – harmless skin lesions occurring in adulthood also known as 'age warts'

Spongiosis – a histopathological term meaning intercellular oedema between keratinocytes, or cells found in the epidermis

Stenosed – narrowed

Striae – stretchmarks

Syringomas – harmless sweat duct tumours

Telangiectasia – small, superficial, dilated blood vessels

Tuberous sclerosus – rare, multisystem genetic disease characterised by skin lesions and internal tumours

Umbilicated – marked by depressed spots resembling the umbilicus

Vesicle – a fluid-filled sac within the epidermis

Violaceous – of a violet colour

Vitiligo – an autoimmune disease characterised by loss of skin pigment

Vulvovaginitis – inflammation of the vagina and vulva

The Basics

Patients with vulval problems have often spent many years in fruitless pursuit of a diagnosis and effective treatment. The reasons for this are as follows:

- Most vulval conditions are chronic dermatological diseases that cannot be cured and must therefore be managed. Such conditions on the vulva often look and behave differently from the same conditions on other parts of the skin; furthermore, management strategies must often be modified in order to be effective on the vulva.
- Dermatological disease of the vulva has far more importance for the patient than the same disease on less emotionally significant areas of the body. Patients frequently present not with symptoms of the vulval disease but with its sexual or relationship consequences. It is therefore no wonder that in the past women with vulval disorders have been unfairly labelled as 'psychosomatic'.
- The vulva and vagina are in the centre of the lower pelvis, are closely related to other pelvic organs and are bound to them by the myofascial structure of the pelvic floor (see Figures 1.1–1.3). Referred vulval pain from other pelvic viscera, and even from the spine and hip joints, is therefore an important concept in understanding vulvovaginal disorders.
- Vulval disease comes with a significant emotional overlay. Embarrassment commonly prevents patients from seeking help. Doctors are only human, and embarrassment can affect them too. Frequently, we hear from patients that they were given a prescription without being examined. It is often difficult for doctors to elicit an adequate history because of the intimate nature of a woman's symptoms and the need to take a detailed sexual and environmental history. Eliciting such histories takes patience and empathy. Patients may either avoid saying what is really on their mind or, alternatively, pour out huge amounts of disorganised, emotionally charged information. It is essential to help them to organise their thoughts. Start at the beginning and get them to think back on how their complaint evolved and how they came to be in your consulting room.

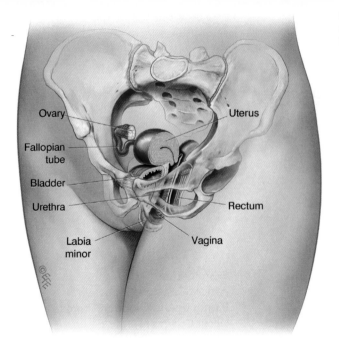

Figure 1.1 The female reproductive tract. With permission from Dr Levent Efe, CMI.

Ovary

Uterus

Fallopian tube

Bladder

Urethra

Rectum

Labia minor

Vagina

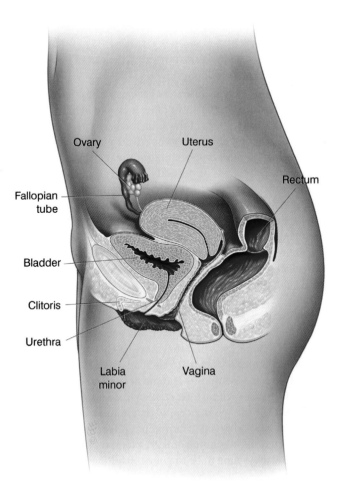

Figure 1.2 The female reproductive tract: side view. With permission from Dr Levent Efe, CMI.

Ovary

Uterus

Fallopian tube

Rectum

Bladder

Clitoris

Urethra

Labia minor

Vagina

(a)

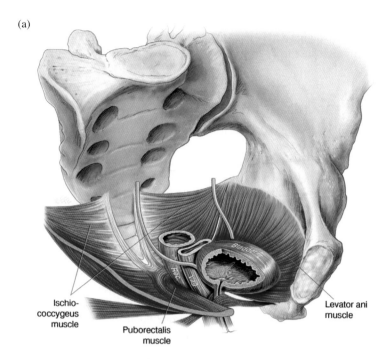

Ischio-
coccygeus
muscle

Puborectalis
muscle

Levator ani
muscle

(b)

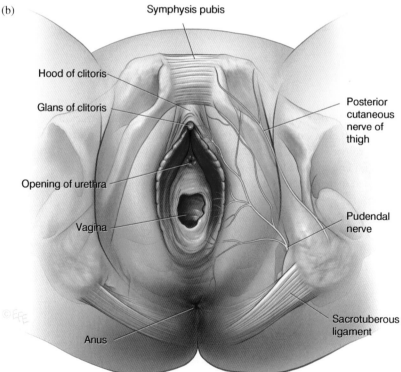

Symphysis pubis

Hood of clitoris

Glans of clitoris

Opening of urethra

Vagina

Anus

Posterior
cutaneous
nerve of
thigh

Pudendal
nerve

Sacrotuberous
ligament

Figure 1.3 (a) The pelvic floor. (b) View of the vulval area. With permission from Dr Levent Efe, CMI.

An emerging issue in the management of vulval disease is the transgender patient. Male-to-female patients with a neovagina and female-to-male patients who have retained a vagina that has been changed by exposure to androgen form a unique group with their own special needs.

Understanding Vulval Conditions

The management of patients with vulval disease fundamentally requires an understanding of dermatological diagnosis and therapy, especially those skin diseases with a predilection for this part of the body. However, dermatological knowledge is not enough. An understanding of gynaecology, gastroenterology, urology, vaginal bacteriology, spinal function and dysfunction, and finally sexual medicine are all essential for optimal management.

Another challenge is the group of patients who appear to defy diagnosis. We believe that this group is very small indeed and that it is possible to classify virtually all patients. However, achieving this relies on very thorough history taking and on combining many different medical disciplines. The more difficult vulval cases are always multifactorial. The term 'vulvodynia' (vulval pain of unknown origin) is not used in this book, as we believe that a rational diagnosis can eventually be found for almost all vulval symptoms.

The purpose of this handbook is to introduce these concepts and to provide practical management recommendations. These are based on our 50 years of collective experience of helping patients with vulval disease, as well as published research by ourselves and others.

We hope this book will give clinicians the tools to approach vulval patients with confidence, and that this will in turn improve the lives of many women.

Anatomy

The Vulva

The vulva is not only part of the skin but is also the entrance to the genital tract. It is essential to understand that vulval skin extends all the way into the hymen. This means that rashes within the vaginal introitus are still classified as vulval, and the patient must be instructed to apply any treatment far enough inside to adequately control these rashes.

The vulva is exposed to many potential irritants, which can result in dermatological symptoms. These include:

- Vaginal discharge, both normal and abnormal
- Menstrual fluid
- Semen
- Urine
- Faeces
- Sweat
- Tight clothes
- Lubricants
- Perfumed products including toilet paper, wet wipes and feminine hygiene products
- Medications
- Pads and panty liners
- Hair-removal practices

The Vagina

The vagina is the conduit between the uterus and the vulva. Its mucosa is prone to similar diseases as in the mouth. Located in the middle of the lower pelvis (see Figure 1.1), its anatomical relationships include the following:

- Bladder and urethra
- Cervix
- Rectum and anus
- Uterovesical and rectovaginal peritoneal pouches
- Sacrum and coccyx

The Pelvic Floor

The pelvic floor is a myofascial structure that encompasses the entire pelvis (Figure 1.3). It is divided functionally into upper and lower parts. The upper part supports the bladder neck, cervix and upper rectum. The lower part supports the urethra, vagina, lower rectum and anus.

The pelvic floor acts as a conduit for pain referral throughout the pelvis. It is closely related to the muscles of the lower back and hip, and may be involved in lumbosacral dysfunction.

Innervation

The innervation of the lower vagina, vulva and anus is from sacral nerve roots S2, S3 and S4 via the pudendal nerve. The anterior vulva is supplied by the genital branch of the genitofemoral nerve (L1–L2) and the ilioinguinal nerve (L1). Thus, lumbosacral, coccygeal and even lower thoracic spinal disorders may produce referred vulval pain.

Clinical Presentation

The majority of patients presenting with chronic vulval symptoms have a skin disease such as eczema, psoriasis or lichen sclerosus, or are suffering from chronic vulvovaginal candidiasis. Many will have a personal or family history of the same condition or will have evidence of it elsewhere on their skin. Patients with eczema are usually atopic. This historical information can provide very helpful clues to a possible diagnosis.

When a patient presents with a vulval complaint, she usually complains of one or more of the following symptoms. Patients sometimes have trouble communicating their thoughts. It can be helpful to run through this list with them, in order to better delineate their real story:

- Itch
- Pre-menstrual or post-menstrual exacerbation of symptoms
- Irritation
- Soreness
- Pain
- Dyspareunia
- Burning
- Stinging
- Stabbing
- Crawling sensations (formication)

- Awareness of the vulva
- Dysuria

The duration of symptoms, any precipitating and exacerbating factors, and previous treatments should be recorded. Bladder, menstrual and bowel function also need to be recorded, as vulvovaginal disease is frequently associated with dysfunction in these systems. Spinal and hip joint disease and dysfunction in voiding may play a significant role in vulval symptoms and should be recorded.

What Do the Symptoms Mean?

Itch and *irritation* are usually due to a non-eroded inflammatory skin condition. *Burning, stinging, stabbing, formication* and *vulval awareness* are usually due to a neuromuscular dysfunction. *Soreness* and *pain* are often due to erosions or fissures, either part of a skin condition or secondary to excoriations produced by scratching.

Dyspareunia

Dyspareunia means pain with sexual intercourse. It is categorised into abdominal and vulvovaginal types. *Abdominal dyspareunia* usually relates to disease or dysfunction at or above the level of the cervix. The pain is experienced in the lower abdomen, as it relates to the upper pelvic floor. *Vulvovaginal dyspareunia* is caused by disease or dysfunction at the level of the lower pelvic floor. The pain is experienced at the vaginal entrance, or further up the vagina. This pain usually relates to a vulvovaginal skin condition, which produces vulval or introital tenderness, splitting or fissuring. It can also relate to dysfunction of the pelvic floor.

Important points to elicit in a history of dyspareunia are:

- Site of entry (or vaginal) dyspareunia (with a mirror if necessary)
- Onset of pain:
  - with foreplay (or masturbation)
  - during vaginal intercourse, or
  - after intercourse is concluded, and
  - whether gradual or sudden

- Duration of pain after intercourse
- Nature of the pain: tearing or splitting, dull or sharp
- What relieves the pain
- Whether the pain is severe enough to result in apareunia
- If the pain is experienced also in a non-sexual context, particularly on tampon insertion or with pressure on the vulva, for example when riding a bicycle

History Taking

The Dermatological History

The following factors in a patient's dermatological history may be relevant to the vulva:

- Atopic disease: eczema, hay fever, asthma
- Psoriasis
- Autoimmune conditions: systemic lupus erythematosus, Sjogren's syndrome, autoimmune thyroiditis, pernicious anaemia

- Allergic reactions to drugs or topical therapy
- Lichen planus

The Gynaecological History

Menstrual disturbance often results in more frequent use of menstrual protection, leading to more contact irritation.

Oestrogen status is important. It is low in post-menopausal and lactating women, and of course in pre-pubertal girls. In general, vaginal candidiasis does not occur in a low-oestrogen environment, and so a post-menopausal woman who does not use systemic or vaginal oestrogen should be assumed not to have candidiasis, unless proven otherwise.

Gynaecological surgery including laser surgery, even of a very minor nature, may cause or worsen vulval disorders.

Patients often assume that their symptoms are due to sexually transmissible infections. It is important to assess this possibility, but the investigation is frequently negative.

Herpes simplex virus infection of the vulva rarely by itself causes chronic vulval symptomatology, but it can be the precipitating factor for chronic vulval dermatitis, entry dyspareunia, neuropathic pain or, very occasionally, anxiety or obsessive–compulsive behaviour.

The Urological History

Urinary incontinence has a strong association with vulval disorders, partly due to simple maceration but also because neuromuscular dysfunction that affects the bladder may also affect the vulva.

Vulvovaginal disorders often result in bladder dysfunction disorders, either infective or non-infective. Many patients, however, will present with the secondary bladder symptoms only, and it will become apparent only after careful history taking that the real culprit is in the vagina or vulva.

Urological surgery, even diagnostic cystoscopy, may cause vulval symptoms.

Very occasionally, symptoms originating from the bladder may be experienced in the vulva and vagina without obvious bladder symptomatology.

The Gastroenterological History

Bowel disturbances, especially diarrhoea, may cause or worsen vulvovaginal disorders.

Haemorrhoids make anal cleansing after defecation more difficult.

Faecal incontinence must always be asked about in women who have had vaginal deliveries. It is surprising how frequently this occurs.

The presence of diseases that produce problems with absorption, most commonly coeliac disease, may result in reduced effectiveness of medications.

Crohn's disease may rarely directly affect the vulva.

The Musculoskeletal History

It is essential to enquire about the following:

- Back injuries (motor vehicle accidents, falls onto the coccyx, heavy lifting, falls causing back injury)
- Sciatica
- Hip joint pain, arthritis and injury

- Lumbosacral osteoarthritis with/without disc protrusion
- Spinal surgery
- Exercise routines
- Weight gain

The Environmental History: Secret Women's Business

It is very likely that your patient has her personal hygiene beliefs, practices and rituals. These are often cherished and difficult to change. You need to find out and you will not unless you ask. Ask specifically about possible irritants and allergens including:

- Washing routines: frequency, use of soap, bubble baths and perfumed oils
- Sanitary pads, incontinence pads, liners and tampons
- Lubricants
- Condoms
- Shaving and waxing
- Douching
- Underwear, G-strings
- Over-the-counter and home remedies
- Exercise routines, including clothing worn
- Sports, particularly cycling and horse riding
- Swimming, saunas and spa baths

The Psychological History

Although this need not be exhaustive, it is important to determine whether:

- The patient is still able to enjoy intercourse
- Her partner is sympathetic
- Her problem has ended any previous sexual relationships
- She is suffering from depression, shame or anxiety independent of, or related to, her problem
- She has had any traumatic sexual experiences, either recently or as a child
- If the patient is a child, sexual abuse has been considered and how has this affected the family
- She has beliefs about her condition that are related to misleading information, often obtained from the internet
- She is angry with the medical profession regarding previous treatment failures

Patient Beliefs

It is important to find out what patients believe is responsible for their symptoms and also their attitude to your possible treatments. Examples of beliefs that may impact on your therapeutic strategies include:

- The assumption that vulval symptoms are due to thrush (although this involves 20% at most)
- Fear that treatment with oestrogen will predispose to breast cancer
- Fear that the use of tampons will result in toxic shock
- A belief that symptoms are due to genital herpes, even when there is no objective evidence

- Fear of the use of any form of corticosteroid (it will 'thin the skin')
- Fear that their skin condition is transmissible
- Fear of cancer
- A belief that their condition is the result of a sexual encounter
- A belief that their condition was transmitted from contact with a fomite (such as a toilet seat)

Summary of History Taking

- Symptoms
- Cycling of symptoms
- Duration of problem
- Previous treatment and whether it has helped, even briefly
- Personal habits
- Dermatological personal and family history
- Atopic disease
- Dyspareunia
- Effect on sexual relationships
- Gynaecological history
- Gastrointestinal history
- Urological history
- General medical history
- Psychological history
- Medications including over-the-counter ones
- Allergies
- Secret women's business

Examination

The vulva and vagina display a high level of anatomical and colour variation. Some of this is congenital, some is age related and much is due to vaginal childbirth. Female genital mutilation will present from time to time, and there is also the increasingly common phenomenon of cosmetic reduction labioplasty. The clinician's ability to define what is 'normal' on examination will therefore be determined by their clinical experience in women's medicine.

Although most vulval problems are fundamentally dermatological, the typical appearance of most skin diseases is very different when they occur on genital skin, and may be quite subtle. A good light and adequate access to the genital skin by careful patient positioning is essential. A couch with foot rests is ideal; however, many patients are humiliated and stressed by having their feet placed in stirrups, and the latter is not necessary for an adequate vulval examination.

Inspect the groin and pubic area first, then the external labia majora, the inter-labial sulcae, and then the vaginal introitus. The clitoral hood should be gently retracted to inspect the glans clitoris. Include the perianal area and natal cleft with your patient lying on her side. It may then be helpful to perform a general skin examination to look for clues that will help with diagnosis, for example with possible psoriasis or lichen planus. Include the buccal mucosa, as this may give a clue to lichen planus.

It is very helpful to use a hand mirror to allow the patient to demonstrate the area of her concern, and so that the clinician can show the patient the areas that actually require application of any topical treatments. Many women have never inspected their own vulva, and it is important to familiarise them with their own anatomy and what the various parts are called.

Common Variations of the Vulva

Common variations of the vulva include:

- Pigmentation: non-Caucasians commonly demonstrate hyperpigmentation of the labia minora; however, patients of all races may develop vulval 'freckling'
- Size of the labia minora: pre-pubertal girls have very small labia minora, but virtually all normal adult pre-menopausal women possess labia minora; after the menopause, these may reduce significantly in size
- Asymmetry of the labia minora
- Size of vaginal opening
- Degree of rugosity of the mucosal surface of the labia minora and vaginal mucosa
- Vulval papillomatosis (tiny projections from the inner surface of the labia minora, a normal variant)
- Prominence of sebaceous glands ('Fordyce spots')
- Erythema: in some patients the sulcus between the labia minora and majora is persistently red in the absence of any pathology
- Length and density of pubic hair
- Clitoral size
- Prominence of gland openings (these may form obvious pits on the mucosal surface)
- Amount of normal discharge
- Apparent webbing at the base of the fourchette

Finding Abnormalities During the Physical Examination

Vulval rashes can be subtle, and initial examination may suggest a normal vulva. Look carefully for:

- Increased erythema of the labia minora, or the sulcus between the labia minora and majora
- Fissuring (skin splits): you may have to gently stretch the skin to find these
- Textural change: lichenification of labia majora and perianal skin, 'cigarette paper wrinkling'
- Evidence of erosions or ulcers
- Mucosal petechiae
- Colour change: light or dark
- Atrophy of mucosa
- Presence of any unusual lesions

Do not be surprised if there are no abnormalities. Many patients with significant vulval symptoms are normal on examination. This finding means that either they have a skin disease that is episodic or that their symptoms are not caused by a dermatological problem.

The Speculum Examination

Many vulval skin diseases involve the vulva only, and there is no need for a speculum examination. The diseases that do extend into the vagina are often so uncomfortable that speculum examination is very difficult and may need to be postponed until their pain has settled with treatment.

If when you examine the vulva the introitus is involved and there appears to be extension into the vagina, attempt a speculum examination using a small, straight-bladed instrument. Remember, you are not taking a Pap smear, and therefore a complete view of the entire vagina is not essential. Your aim is to visualise enough of the vaginal wall to determine the degree of intra-vaginal inflammation.

Look for:
- Erythema, and whether it is confluent or patchy
- Erosions
- Petechiae
- Degree, colour and type of discharge

Investigations

The most commonly performed investigations in patients with vulval disease are:
- Low vaginal swab for bacterial or *Candida* infection
- Viral swab for PCR of herpes simplex virus if suspected; this must be taken from an ulcer or erosion
- Vulval swab for bacterial or *Candida* infection
- Scraping of vulval skin for dermatophyte (tinea) infection
- Skin biopsy

All patients should have a low vaginal swab. A high vaginal swab taken during a speculum examination is unnecessary and may not reflect the environment of the lower vagina. Furthermore, passing a speculum past inflamed vulval skin is often exquisitely painful.

A vulval swab and scraping is performed if infection of the hair-bearing skin is suspected clinically.

A skin biopsy is performed if there is a visible rash or lesion that is diagnosable by biopsy, particularly suspected malignancy. It should never be performed on clinically normal skin.

Other tests that may be relevant include:
- Mid-stream urine if urological symptoms are present
- Patch testing if contact allergy is suspected
- Follicle-stimulating hormone: this may in some cases be required to assist in confirming menopause
- Tests for systemic autoimmune disease, which may be relevant in patients with conditions such as lichen sclerosus

Colposcopy is usually unnecessary in the diagnosis of vulvovaginal disorders, except when vulval intra-epithelial neoplasia is suspected. The use of acetic acid on the vulva is unnecessary in benign skin diseases and usually produces significant stinging, which patients find traumatic.

Patient Categorisation

At the end of your history taking and examination, you will find that patients with vulval disease fall into the following broad categories:

- Patients with a rash and non-cycling symptoms
- Patients with a rash and cyclical symptoms
- Patients with a rash or lesion and no symptoms
- Patients with no rash but symptoms

This will be discussed in more detail later in the book.

Summing Up: Common Things Occur Commonly

The majority of patients presenting with chronic vulval symptoms have a vulval presentation of a common skin disease such as eczema, psoriasis or lichen sclerosus, or are suffering from chronic vulvovaginal candidiasis. Many will have a personal or family history of the same condition elsewhere on the skin. Many patients with eczema are atopic. This historical information can provide very helpful clues to a possible diagnosis.

Chapter 2

Using Topical Corticosteroids on the Vulva

Topical corticosteroids on the vulva are very safe if used properly and supervised regularly. We provide a guide to the safe and effective use of these essential drugs.

Topical corticosteroids are a dermatological therapeutic mainstay. They are appropriate in the treatment of virtually all inflammatory dermatoses everywhere on the skin, and on the vulva, which is part of the skin.

They are used in different ways in different situations and, if used appropriately and correctly, they are very safe. For instance, in lichen sclerosus and lichen planus, they are used continuously, but in psoriasis and dermatitis they are used intermittently, first for initial treatment and then for flare-ups. Details of how to treat these conditions are found in the appropriate chapters.

These time-tested medications, which have been available for over 60 years, have been much maligned in the last 15 years. So-called 'corticosteroid phobia' has resulted in doctors and patients being too scared to use them adequately; this then denies patients the right sort of treatment that will greatly improve their quality of life.

In general, the following principles will keep your patients safe:

- Use ointment bases in preference to creams. Ointments adhere better to genital skin, and creams contain preservatives that may sting. This does not suit all patients, but it suits most.
- Make sure your diagnosis is right, i.e. your patient has a corticosteroid-responsive dermatosis. If you use topical corticosteroids to treat an infection such as tinea, you will make the situation worse, not better.
- Know your corticosteroid potencies – see Table 2.1.
- Titrate the dose of your treatment to the severity of the condition you are treating. If it is mild, you can use the moderate to weak preparations. If severe, use potent ones. If very severe, use super-potent preparations.
- Start strong and work down.
- Be aware that clobetasol propionate is super-potent and therefore is much easier to get into trouble with than weaker preparations. It is mentioned in many publications on vulval disease but is only one of many topical corticosteroids available, and in many situations it is not the best.
- Do not use time as a guideline for how long you treat – use clinical response. One of the biggest mistakes made by clinicians is under-treatment. Your patient's skin should be back to subjective and objective normality before your reduce.

Table 2.1 Topical corticosteroids

Potency class	Generic name	Comments
Mild	Hydrocortisone 1–2%	Useful in dermatitis, psoriasis and maintenance treatment of lichen sclerosus
Moderate	Triamcinolone 0.2–0.25%	Useful in dermatitis, psoriasis and maintenance treatment of lichen sclerosus
	Aclometasone dipropionate 0.05%	
	Clobetasone butyrate 0.05%	
	Methylprednisolone aceponate 0.1%	
	Desonide 0.05%	
	Betamethasone valerate 0.02%	
Potent	Mometasone furoate 0.1%	Useful for initial treatment of all inflammatory dermatoses but in general not for very long-term use outside of lichen planus
	Triamcinolone acetonide 0.05–1.0%	
	Betamethasone dipropionate 0.05%	
	Betamethasone valerate 0.05–1.0%	
Super-potent	Clobetasol propionate 0.05%	Take care! Only for severe lichen sclerosus, lichen planus and very lichenified dermatitis. Monitor carefully
	Halobetasol propionate 0.05%	Same precautions as for clobetasol propionate

- Get your patient used to the fact that it is OK to use topical corticosteroids long term. Most vulval dermatoses are chronic and need ongoing treatment. Perianal skin is less tolerant of topical corticosteroids than the vulva. In general, you should use weaker preparations there.
- Avoid combination products containing antibiotics or antifungals. Long-term use can result in sensitisation.
- It is rare to be genuinely allergic to topical corticosteroids, but it does happen. If your patient starts off doing well but subsequently stops improving or becomes worse, consider this possibility.
- The use of topical corticosteroids on the small area involved in treating vulval disease will not result in absorption that could cause any systemic side effects. The area is less than 1% of the total body surface.
- The commonest side effect is redness. This always gets better with a reduction in corticosteroid dose.
- As long as you are following these rules, atrophy is most unlikely.
- Occasionally, you may produce telangiectasia, and in small girls, even early pubic hair. Does this really matter when the patient is getting better?
- Do not think you can substitute calcineurin inhibitors such as pimecrolimus and tacrolimus for topical corticosteroids, or that you should use them just because they aren't 'steroids'. They are expensive, they sting and we do not know what they might do to patients in the very long term as we have less than 20 years' experience with them.
- Do not be scared of topical corticosteroids. Embrace them!

Table 2.1 gives you a selection of topical corticosteroids to use in your practice. This list is by no means exhaustive but sets out the medications that we have had personal experience with and have found to be reasonably affordable and useful. Not all of them are available in every country. Remember that the percentage on the tube does not necessarily indicate that the product is more or less potent.

If you live in a country where you are able to access methylprednisolone aceponate and/or aclometasone dipropionate 0.05%, we find these particularly well tolerated and unlikely to produce any side effects, even with very long term use.

Chapter 3

Red Vulval Rashes

The most common presentation of a vulval skin problem is an itchy red rash. This group includes inflammatory dermatoses, infections, hypersensitivity reactions and one malignancy.

Dermatitis, psoriasis and chronic vulvovaginal candidiasis are all very common causes of red, itchy rashes with variable degrees of scaling. Corticosteroid-induced dermatitis occurs when moderate to potent topical corticosteroid is used for long periods of time and is encountered most often in patients requiring this treatment for other dermatoses such as lichen sclerosus and lichen planus. Tinea is uncommon, and extra-mammary Paget's disease and oestrogen-hypersensitivity vulvovaginitis are rare.

On first sight, all these conditions look much the same. A combination of history taking, investigation and response to therapy will ultimately enable a diagnosis and effective treatment.

Dermatitis

Dermatitis is the most common cause of chronic vulval symptoms, usually dominated by itch. There are two forms: endogenous and exogenous.

Endogenous dermatitis (or eczema) describes a number of inflammatory dermatoses that are intrinsic to the patient. The majority of patients with endogenous vulval dermatitis are atopic, and their condition is a localised form of atopic dermatitis. History taking often reveals asthma, hay fever or dermatitis on other parts of the skin, or a strong family history of atopy.

Exogenous dermatitis describes an inflammatory skin disease caused by exogenous agents: allergens and irritants.

All forms of dermatitis have in common a histological appearance known as 'spongiosis'. Under the microscope, spongiosis represents oedema of the epidermal layer of the skin, so that individual cells are separated by oedema fluid. 'Spongiotic dermatitis' is therefore a term that is commonly used by pathologists when describing dermatitis.

The forms of endogenous dermatitis that involve the vulva are:

- Atopic dermatitis
- Seborrhoeic dermatitis

The forms of exogenous dermatitis that involve the vulva are:

- Irritant contact dermatitis
- Allergic contact dermatitis

The following conditions, which will be discussed below, resemble chronic dermatitis but have unique characteristics:

- Chronic vulvovaginal candidiasis
- Oestrogen-hypersensitivity vulvovaginitis
- Corticosteroid-induced dermatitis (periorificial dermatitis)

Presentation

Patients with dermatitis are almost always itchy, but if the mucosal surface is involved, they will also experience burning, and excoriations from scratching and fissures, which are commonly found in all vulval dermatoses, will produce pain and dyspareunia.

The symptoms are normally worse at night and interfere with sleep. Clothes and activities that increase heat, sweat and friction often exacerbate dermatitis.

Examination

Examination shows poorly defined erythema of the labia and perineum that may extend onto the mons pubis and the inner thighs. In long-standing cases, lichenification is common, resulting in rugosity of the labia majora and perianal skin. The vestibule is erythematous, and there may be white plaques present on the mucosal surfaces and labia.

Close examination often reveals fissuring, particularly around the introitus or in the inter-labial clefts. The vagina is not involved, and there is no discharge unless superinfection is present. Patients with dermatitis may report an offensive discharge, but this is actually desquamation. This tends to remit when the dermatitis is controlled. If the vaginal culture shows *Candida albicans*, then this requires treatment in addition to the dermatitis.

Occasionally, bacterial superinfection with *Staphylococcus aureus* or *Streptococcus pyogenes* can occur in vulval dermatitis, as in dermatitis on any other part of the skin. This may present as a cellulitis, giving a typical oedematous appearance; however, weeping and crusting, known as impetiginisation, may also be a sign. This is treated with an appropriate oral antibiotic. Our experience has shown that group B *Streptococcus* isolates from the vagina are not relevant to vulvovaginal pathology and should be ignored

Atopic Dermatitis

An example of atopic dermatitis is shown in Figure 3.1. Most patients with vulval dermatitis are atopic. They may have a current or past history of atopic dermatitis on other parts of their skin, or of asthma or hay fever.

The distribution of the rash includes the labia majora and minora and perineum. The perianal area may also be involved but not the vagina.

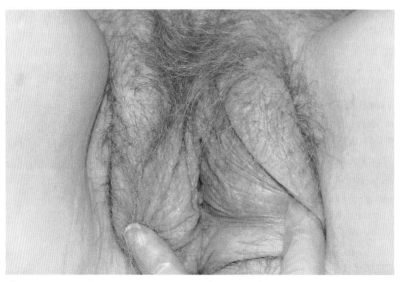

Figure 3.1 Atopic dermatitis. Note excoriations due to scratching.

Atopic patients are typically intolerant of irritants. They are unable to use soap or wear occlusive clothing without discomfort.

Atopic dermatitis of the vulva may occur at any age. It usually responds readily to simple management (see 'Management' below). Very occasionally, patients with severe lichenification may be treatment resistant.

Post-menopausal women may experience vulval atopic dermatitis for the first time in connection with oestrogen deficiency. They may suffer not only from vaginal dryness but also from itching of the labia. In this group where incontinence of urine is not uncommon, maceration from the incontinence itself and also from the wearing of pads exacerbates the problem.

In children, atopic dermatitis of the vulva has a somewhat different set of irritants and triggers related to sporting activities such as ballet (nylon tights) and swimming lessons (chlorinated water, wet swimming costumes), bubble bath or using shampoo in the bath, sand from a sandpit, maceration from nappies (diapers) and pull-ups, dysfunctional voiding leading to chronic maceration and faecal incontinence from chronic constipation.

Seborrhoeic Dermatitis

Seborrhoeic dermatitis is very common as a cause of dandruff, but it is relatively uncommon as a cause of vulvitis. Such patients are not atopic but do have chronic problems with an itchy, scaly scalp and sometimes rashes on the central chest and in the axilla.

It can be differentiated from atopic dermatitis by the involvement of other typical sites such as the scalp and axilla, as well as a negative history of atopy.

In vulval seborrhoeic dermatitis, the extent of the rash is often greater than with atopic dermatitis, with the rash extending into the inguinal folds, inner thighs and mons pubis. There is a characteristically greasy, scaly surface. The vagina is not involved.

Seborrhoeic dermatitis tends to be less itchy than atopic dermatitis. It is a very chronic condition that tends to be exacerbated at times of stress.

The cause of seborrhoeic dermatitis is unknown, but in some patients it is thought that the presence of *Malassezia* sp. yeast on the skin is a trigger. For this reason some patients benefit from the use of antifungal creams in addition to topical corticosteroids.

Irritant Contact Dermatitis

Vulval dermatitis due to chronic exogenous irritation presents with a persistent low-grade dermatitis in the area in contact with the irritant. Therefore, in most cases only the labia majora and perineum are involved.

Many patients with this condition are also atopic and are therefore more prone to problems with irritants, so that their dermatitis is a combination of both conditions.

There are some instances where irritant dermatitis is not associated with atopy, and in these cases there is often a severe compromise of the cutaneous barrier. This includes patients who are incontinent of urine and/or faeces, who constantly wear macerated incontinence garments or who are confined to a wheelchair. Such patients are often in nursing homes. They present a very difficult challenge.

Women who engage in intense sporting activities, particularly bicycle riding, may develop a chronic vulvitis from friction, occlusive nylon sports clothes and sweating. In the case of serious cyclists, vulval oedema may become a disabling problem.

Some feminine hygiene products may also cause irritant contact dermatitis, and this includes the use of shower gels, perfumed wipes, sprays, douches and essential oils. Many women feel the need to clean the genital area more thoroughly than other parts of the skin, and unintentionally produce dermatitis in their attempts to feel 'fresh'.

Another common practice that creates problems is the constant use of panty liners. Some women say they feel cleaner if they always wear a liner. Others say they do not feel 'secure' without a liner to shield the opening of their vagina. The occlusion caused by liners, most of which contain a layer of plastic, is a common cause of irritant contact dermatitis.

Tight, occlusive nylon clothes, G-string underwear, pantyhose and control garments can also cause irritation by producing constant friction.

Waxing and other hair-removal products may cause irritation, particularly as hair begins to grow back. It is not uncommon for waxing to be associated with an irritating folliculitis.

The constant use of imidazole antifungal creams on the vulva frequently causes an irritant reaction.

When skin is inflamed, possible irritants will often aggravate the condition, and things that are normally tolerated may begin to cause a problem. Friction from intercourse may become intensely uncomfortable, and contact with semen and saliva may cause burning and stinging.

Allergic Contact Dermatitis

Allergic contact dermatitis (Figure 3.2) results from contact with a true allergen: a substance to which a patient mounts a type IV allergic response resulting in severe, vesicular, eroded dermatitis. Fortunately, it is a rare event.

It can present either as a sudden-onset acute dermatitis or as a chronic non-responsive condition that appears frustratingly resistant to treatment. Because of the severity of the allergic reaction, pain and soreness is often more of a feature than itch. It often extends to the skin outside the area of direct contact and may be found in other places such as the fingers or eyelids as a result of accidentally transferring the allergen.

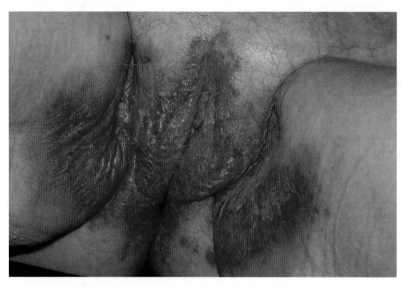

Figure 3.2 Allergic contact dermatitis.

The most common cause of allergic contact dermatitis of the vulva is medications, both prescribed and over the counter. These include azole antifungal creams, oestrogen creams, antibiotics, products containing tea-tree oil, topical anaesthetics particularly benzocaine, other vaginal creams and topical corticosteroids. The latter are particularly difficult to identify as the cortisone both causes an allergic reaction and suppresses it simultaneously. Compounded products containing amitriptyline may also cause allergic contact dermatitis.

When moisturisers, lubricants, sanitary pads and toilet paper cause an allergic contact dermatitis, the culprit is usually the perfumes and preservatives in these products.

The use of wet wipes containing the preservative methylisothiazolinone has become a world-wide phenomenon in causing contact dermatitis of the genital region in both adults and children.

Latex in condoms may cause allergy. Polyurethane condoms are non-allergenic and may be substituted.

When vulval dermatitis is of sudden onset, severe and related to the use of a new product, suspect allergic contact dermatitis. It is also a diagnostic possibility in recalcitrant or severe cases of dermatitis. The allergen is identified by patch testing, a painstaking and subspecialised process that requires referral to a dermatologist.

In rare cases, seminal fluid may cause true contact allergic reaction. Patients who suffer from this experience severe irritation when their partner ejaculates. This is followed by persistent vulval and vaginal dermatitis. Many of them discover for themselves that condoms protect them, and this history is a clue to the nature of the problem. A confounder, however, is that seminal fluid can be irritating to an already inflamed vagina without true allergy. If a patient gives this history, referral to a dermatologist is recommended.

Corticosteroid-Induced Dermatitis

Corticosteroid-induced dermatitis (Figure 3.3), also known as periorificial dermatitis, is not a true dermatitis but a side effect of the use of potent corticosteroids on the vulva. It usually

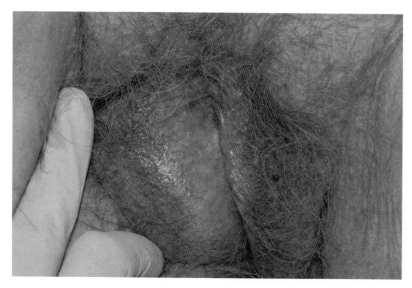

Figure 3.3 Corticosteroid-induced dermatitis.

occurs when patients use potent, fluorinated corticosteroids continually for long periods of time and is very unlikely with weak corticosteroids, even when these are used chronically. Patients complain that, although their condition is not well controlled with their medication, any attempt to withdraw it results in even more severe symptoms.

The labia majora and minora become erythematous or even violaceous. Telangiectasia may appear, and skin fragility may result in fissuring and tearing during intercourse. Patients commonly complain of a constant burning sensation. Pustules and papules can occur, but scaling is not present.

It is important to recognise this symptom as a side effect of corticosteroid. If it is not differentiated from ordinary dermatitis, there is a risk that even stronger preparations will be used, which will exacerbate the condition.

Corticosteroid-induced dermatitis is treated by the gradual withdrawal of the potent corticosteroid, reducing to moderate and then weak products. The withdrawal process may be difficult, and patients often experience an exacerbation of burning and itching as the strength of the medication reduces. The process commonly takes 6 weeks. Oral doxy-cycline reduces the symptoms and is usually given for the entire 6-week period at a dose of 50–100 mg/day.

Although corticosteroid-induced dermatitis can be difficult to treat initially, it is a completely reversible condition. It is important to be able to reassure patients about this, as fear of corticosteroids is widespread and is a major barrier to effective treatment compliance.

Management

By the time a patient presents with vulval dermatitis, she has often developed one or more secondary problems. The most common of these is dyspareunia, the management of which is discussed in Chapter 8. The first step in management is control of the dermatitis before dealing with secondary issues.

The principles of treating vulval dermatitis include:

- Environmental modification, which includes eradication of irritant substances
- Diagnosis and treatment of superinfection
- Identification of possible allergens
- Use of topical corticosteroids
- Alternatives to topical corticosteroids
- Management of secondary dyspareunia

Environmental Modification

Topical corticosteroids alone will not substantially improve any form of genital dermatitis. This is because genital skin is exposed to many contact irritants and possibly to allergens. Even in endogenous dermatitis, these local factors exacerbate the clinical problem.

Treatment must start with identifying and managing the causes of an exogenous dermatitis, and the exacerbating factors in an endogenous dermatitis.

Most patients have more than one causative or exacerbating factor. The patient needs to understand that significant improvement will not be possible until these factors are controlled.

If you suspect that one of the patient's topical medications or cosmetic products is responsible, stop the use of that product.

Common irritants include:

- Soap
- Bubble bath
- Essential oils
- Sanitary pads and liners
- Prolonged use of antifungal creams
- Lubricants
- Wet wipes
- Douches
- Waxing and shaving products
- Nylon underwear
- Pantyhose
- G-strings
- Tight clothes
- Gym clothes
- Friction from bicycle seats

Patients should be advised to:

- Use a soap substitute
- Wear cotton underwear
- Use tampons rather than pads
- Substitute a wet cloth for wet wipes (this can be kept in a snap-lock bag)
- Avoid routine use of panty liners
- Discard G-strings
- Stop using antifungal creams
- Discard perfumed products
- Wear loose clothes

- Avoid nylon bike pants and pantyhose
- Avoid activities that cause heavy sweating and/or friction until improved

Dermatitis always involves an element of dryness, so a bland emollient is a necessary part of management and prevention. In general, this should be non-perfumed, non-irritating and of a consistency that is comfortable and acceptable for the patient. We recommend daily use as often as possible. On inflamed skin, many products cause stinging. This is less likely to happen with ointments than creams. It is not an allergy and settles as the skin recovers.

Diagnosis and Treatment of Superinfection

All patients should have a low vaginal swab and a vulval swab. The organisms that may cause superinfection are:

- *Candida albicans* (vagina)
- *Staphylococcus aureus* (vulva)
- *Streptococcus pyogenes* (vulva)

A finding of *C. albicans* has to be interpreted in line with symptoms and signs. It may indicate superinfection in dermatitis, or possibly the independent diagnosis of chronic vulvovaginal candidiasis. If the history is typical of chronic candidiasis, the patient will need prolonged antifungal treatment. A rapid response to a single oral dose of fluconazole 150 mg is the most pragmatic way to determine whether *C. albicans* is partially responsible for the patient's symptoms. This is because, in patients with dermatitis, topical antifungals run the risk of causing irritation.

Bacterial infection is treated with appropriate oral antibiotics, according to antibiotic sensitivities.

It is important to note that a finding of group B or C Streptococcus should be ignored in this situation.

Identification of Possible Allergens

Allergic contact dermatitis is not a common cause of vulvitis but should be suspected when the dermatitis is severe, eroded, refractory to treatment or extends to the inner thighs and lower abdomen.

Possible allergens include:

- Perfumes and preservatives in hygiene products, wet wipes and scented toilet paper
- Topical antifungal and antibiotic creams
- Latex in condoms
- Nail polish
- Semen (these patients invariably realise that semen stings and that their problem is solved by using condoms)
- Topical corticosteroids
- Topical oestrogens
- Lubricants

If allergic contact dermatitis is suspected, the initial examination should include taking a careful history. Patients often do not remember every substance that has been applied to their skin while in the office with you. Ask them to write down everything they can think of that is applied to the vulva.

You will note that a number of products are on both the irritant and the allergen lists. It is common for many substances to irritate but rarer for them to cause a true allergy.

Allergic contact dermatitis is diagnosed by patch testing. Such patients should be referred to a dermatologist. Elimination of the offending substance will solve the problem.

In the case of semen allergy, diagnosis is by skin prick testing and radioallergosor bent testing (RAST). Such patients may be able to be desensitised by an immunologist.

Latex allergy may be diagnosed with specific IgE serology.

Use of Topical Corticosteroids

In general, a weak topical corticosteroid (hydrocortisone 1%) is effective and appropriate in treating all forms of genital dermatitis, provided environmental modification is in place.

The advantage of this weak cortisone is that it can be used for long periods of time without adverse effects. This is essential, as many forms of dermatitis are chronic conditions that require long-term control.

When using a topical corticosteroid on the vulva, ointments are preferable to creams. Creams contain preservatives that may cause stinging, irritation or even frank allergy.

Hydrocortisone 1% ointment applied twice daily for up to 1 month is often all that is necessary to control the inflammation. It may then be used as needed for recurrences.

If lichenification is present, a potent topical corticosteroid ointment may be used safely once daily until this has resolved. This may take as long as a month. As soon as the patient has recovered, the topical corticosteroid should be reduced gradually, first to medium potency for a month and then to hydrocortisone 1%.

Intra-lesional triamcinolone may sometimes be needed for patients with recalcitrant areas of lichen simplex chronicus (white, thickened areas; see Chapter 4).

These warnings about potent topical corticosteroids are not intended to discourage their use. Even with long-term treatment, the weak preparations are safe and appropriate on the vulva. 'Corticosteroid phobia' is common in the community, and patients frequently receive warnings from health professionals about their potential to 'thin the skin'. Such warnings only serve to discourage treatment adherence and deny patients with a genuine problem the treatment they need. In practice, adverse effects of cortisone are seen only with prolonged inappropriate use, and are reversible. As a doctor, it is important to be positive about the use of these products with patients who have a chronic corticosteroid-responsive skin condition.

Alternatives to Topical Corticosteroids

There are very few alternatives to the use of topical corticosteroids when treating dermatitis, particularly where it is severe.

The topical calcineurin inhibitors pimecrolimus 1% and tacrolimus 0.03 and 0.1% may be used to treat vulval dermatitis; however, they are significantly more expensive than topical corticosteroids and both frequently cause stinging. It is usually necessary to gain control of the dermatitis first with a topical corticosteroid before initiating their use.

Some patients prefer not to use a corticosteroid because of adverse publicity about long-term safety. This fear may interfere significantly with compliance. For this reason, long-term maintenance calcineurin inhibitors may have better acceptance by some patients.

Management of Dyspareunia

All forms of vulval dermatitis have a tendency to cause splitting. Itch and subsequent scratching may cause raw areas and excoriation. As a result, intercourse may cause discomfort.

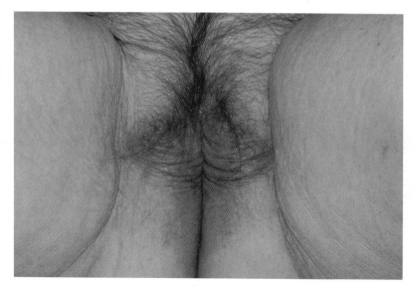

Figure 3.4 Psoriasis. Note the well-demarcated border and symmetry.

In many cases, simple treatment of the underlying condition is all that is required for dyspareunia to resolve. However, in any painful vulval condition, secondary pelvic floor muscle spasm may continue after adequate control of the dermatitis.

If dyspareunia does not resolve after symptoms have been controlled and the vulva has returned to normal objectively, pelvic floor muscle dysfunction should be suspected and treated (see Chapter 8).

Psoriasis

Psoriasis (Figures 3.4–3.6) is also a common vulval condition but less so than dermatitis, with which it is most often confused. Psoriasis of the vulva is easy to diagnose if present elsewhere on the skin, but it can occur solely on genital skin. On the pubic area, it is usually typical with well-defined scaly red plaques, but on the vulva itself, it lacks the scale and sometimes the sharp edge of typical psoriasis. When scale occurs in vulval psoriasis, it is usually in the sulcus between the labia minora and majora.

The lesions are usually more erythematous and well defined than dermatitis, and are usually bilaterally symmetrical, although unilateral lesions are possible. Psoriasis does not involve the vagina, but the labia are usually involved, and the rash can extend inwards as far as the vestibule. The perianal area and natal cleft may be involved, and natal cleft involvement is a useful sign, as it is not seen in dermatitis. Lichenification of the perianal skin and labia majora may be severe.

A search for subtle signs of psoriasis such as nail pitting, scalp scaling, and thickening and scaling of the dorsal surface of the elbows and knees may provide helpful diagnostic clues, as does a family history of psoriasis.

History Taking

The history often gives clues as to whether the problem is psoriasis or eczema. Psoriasis is often episodic in nature, with the episodes not always clearly related to any triggers. Psoriasis

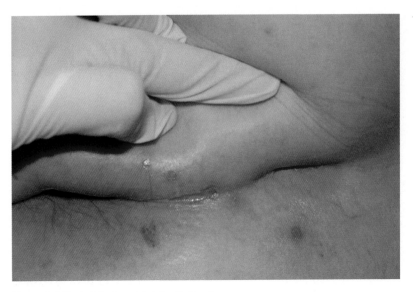

Figure 3.5 Psoriasis in the natal cleft with fissuring.

is classically exacerbated by situational stress or physical illness, particularly streptococcal throat infections. It may also be precipitated by vaginal candidiasis or vaginal surgery. In some cases, psoriasis flares pre-menstrually.

A common history is of a very long-standing itchy vulvitis, present for years and treated intermittently by potent topical corticosteroid with some response but without lasting improvement.

Vulval psoriasis is often itchy. It may become sore if eroded by scratching. It may flare pre-menstrually but this is not invariable.

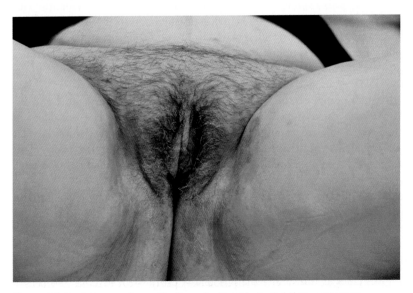

Figure 3.6 Psoriasis, extending out to the groins. Note the typical silvery appearance.

There is no specific diagnostic test for psoriasis. Although a classic histopathology is described, this is often lacking on the vulva and biopsies are often reported as 'non-specific inflammation' or 'spongiotic dermatitis'. Therefore, diagnosis relies on the clinician's judgement and is supported by family history and/or signs of psoriasis elsewhere on the skin.

Management

Psoriasis usually improves initially with topical steroids, but these can lose effectiveness after some weeks. Treatment with topical therapy specific for psoriasis is necessary to continue improvement and maintain control, and the patient should be given a management plan for the inevitable flare-ups.

A diagnosis of psoriasis can be distressing for many patients. The condition is common enough for many people to have heard of it and also to realise that it is not curable and, in a few cases, very severe. It is important to put this in perspective: psoriasis is common, in most cases is not severe, and on the vulva is nearly always able to be controlled with topical therapy.

The same principles of environmental modification and infection control that are used for patients with dermatitis should be put into place.

In the initial stages of treating psoriasis, it is usual for weak topical corticosteroids, which are useful in dermatitis, to be ineffective. A topical medium-potency cortisone ointment is used at night until significant symptomatic and objective improvement is achieved. This often takes at least 4 weeks. As soon as the patient is comfortable and eroded or split areas have healed, add a specific psoriasis treatment such as:

- 2% LPC (liquor picis carbonis – a tar product) in aqueous cream or white soft paraffin
- Calcipotriol 0.5% ointment

These products are applied in the morning and the cortisone is applied at night. Both are effective maintenance preparations for psoriasis. It usually takes several weeks for optimal efficacy to be achieved. Once adequate improvement is achieved, the steroid ointment is ceased and the LPC and/or calcipotriol are continued once or twice daily. Some patients benefit from using both once per day. Long-term management is required on the vulva, and it is important to make sure patients realise this.

Both LPC and calcipotriol should be tested on the cubital fossa for a few days before applying to the vulva to ensure that they do not cause a severe irritant or allergic reaction.

Psoriasis can, like eczema, be complicated by lichenification. In this situation, a potent topical corticosteroid is used to initiate treatment as described above.

Psoriasis can be an unpredictable and frustrating disease for the patient. It is a matter of trial and error to find the ideal maintenance and flare-up regimen. In general, patients fare best when they can combine a non-corticosteroid preventative treatment with intermittent use of topical corticosteroids for flare-ups.

Apart from LPC and calcipotriol, there are a number of other maintenance formulations that can be helpful. Emollients such as Bepanthen® ointment, Amolin® cream, or zinc and castor oil give many patients relief. Topical calcineurin inhibitors such as pimecrolimus 1% or tacrolimus 0.03 or 0.1% may be helpful but can cause unacceptable stinging, as in dermatitis. It is important to remember that many psoriasis patients have unpredictable reactions to various preparations. Prolonged burning and stinging after using one treatment means that it should be discontinued and another tried.

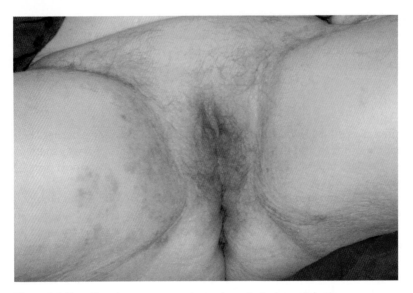

Figure 3.7 Tinea. Note the asymmetry and extension onto the lower abdomen.

If there is co-existent candidiasis, prolonged antifungal treatment is essential until the psoriasis is well controlled. This is because many cases of psoriasis are driven by chronic candidiasis.

Genital psoriasis not able to be controlled by topical therapy may require more advanced treatments such as narrowband UVB phototherapy or systemic medication. In this very uncommon situation, referral to a dermatologist is recommended.

Tinea

This very common fungal infection (Figure 3.7) is in fact an uncommon cause of vulval disease. It is caused by the same dermatophyte fungi that are responsible for tinea pedis and other types of tinea.

Presentation

Patients present with an itchy, scaly bilateral or unilateral rash involving the labia majora, which may extend to both inguinal folds and lower abdomen. The edge is usually better demarcated than in dermatitis, and it is often less symmetrical. It may be difficult to differentiate clinically from psoriasis or dermatitis but is worsened by topical corticosteroid treatment, even if there is temporary improvement at first.

Rarely, vulval tinea may present with pustules and nodules and may closely simulate boils or hidradenitis suppurativa.

Investigation

A fungal skin scraping or biopsy is essential to make a diagnosis.

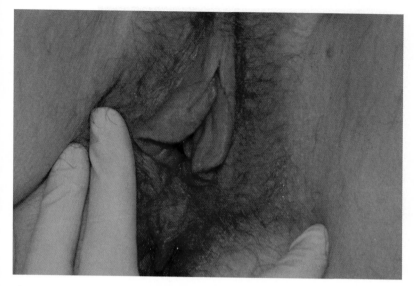

Figure 3.8 Chronic vulvovaginal candidiasis. Note the oedematous rash extending out to the hair-bearing surface of the labia majora. The external border is poorly demarcated.

Management

Most cases of vulval tinea require oral antifungal treatment for two reasons:

1. The hair follicles are involved.
2. There is almost invariably foot involvement with the same fungus and unless this is adequately treated the patient runs the risk of re-inoculating herself.

The following antifungal medications may be used for tinea:

- Griseofulvin 500 mg/day
- Terbinafine 250 mg/day
- Fluconazole 150 mg/week
- Itraconazole 200 mg daily for 1 week repeating monthly

Each needs to be given until there is complete clearance of the rash on the vulva and the feet (if present), and a repeat scraping is negative. The minimum duration of treatment is typically 4–6 weeks; however, longer treatment periods may be required.

For patients who are unwilling to take oral medication, topical terbinafine will control symptoms. It should be used daily for several weeks. Relapse is common when it is stopped.

Chronic Vulvovaginal Candidiasis

Approximately 20% of women carry *Candida* yeast (the majority *C. albicans* and about 5% *C. glabrata*) in the vagina, but only a small number suffer from recurrent or chronic candidiasis (Figures 3.8 and 3.9).

Acute candidiasis is well understood and easily recognised and treated; however, patients with the chronic form of vulvovaginal candidiasis are a much less well recognised and managed group. The condition may start at any age, from menarche onwards. It ceases at

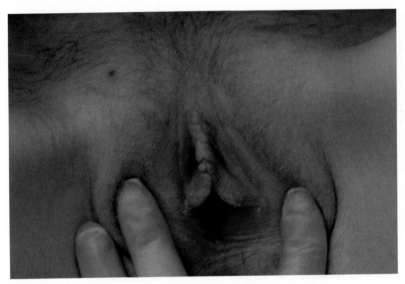

Figure 3.9 Chronic vulvovaginal candidiasis. Note the associated inter-labial rash with fissuring.

menopause provided oestrogen-replacement therapy is not used. Vulvovaginal candidiasis is oestrogen dependent and in healthy women, does not occur in its absence.

Recurrent vulvovaginal candidiasis is defined as four or more attacks of vulvovaginal candidiasis proven microbiologically per year. Chronic vulvovaginal candidiasis is defined as patients who are constantly symptomatic, and has recently been formally described.

Presentation

Chronic vulvovaginal candidiasis presents with recurrent or constant itch, but dyspareunia, soreness, burning, swelling, fissuring and pain are common. It is characteristic but not invariable for these symptoms to cycle, being most severe in the pre-menstrual week and suddenly improving on the first day of menstruation.

Discharge is common but may be absent, and the typical cheesy exudate of acute candidiasis is not seen. It is typical for courses of oral antibiotics to exacerbate or precipitate symptoms.

The patient's partner may experience post-coital itching and penile rash, which is also characteristic, but is present in only a minority. Patients often give a history of response to topical and oral antifungals; however, recurrence of symptoms is the rule when they are ceased. There may also be a history of worsening symptoms with the use of potent topical steroids. As most patients do benefit to some extent from antifungal medications, they use them frequently, and as a result vaginal cultures may return a false negative. Therefore, a negative swab does not rule out this condition, particularly if other aspects of the history are present.

Many patients can recall recurrent attacks of acute candidiasis from adolescence onwards. They state that initially such attacks responded to topical antifungal medication but, with time, resistance to topical therapy occurred, attacks became more frequent and eventually symptoms became constant.

Chronic vulvovaginal candidiasis can be a very difficult diagnosis. A trial of prolonged antifungal therapy is indicated if your patient has the following:

- A persistent non-erosive vulvovaginitis that cycles, being most severe in the pre-menstrual week
- A vulvovaginitis that has responded previously (even if only briefly) to topical or oral antifungals
- Previous positive swabs for *Candida* sp. even if this has been inconsistent and is not positive on *this* occasion
- A history of exacerbation as a result of taking antibiotics

Such a trial often becomes the ultimate diagnostic test.

The rash in this condition may vary from no apparent abnormality to severe erythema, involving the whole vulva and perianal area, and vagina, with varying degrees of oedema and fissuring on the perineum and inter-labial sulcus. The most typical presentation, however, is a vulvovaginitis with erythema of the labia minora extending into the sulcus between the labia minora and majora.

Investigation

When taking the swab, the yield is best from a low rather than a high vaginal swab. If the typical history is present, any degree of culture positivity is significant. Commonly, false negatives occur, possibly due to the fact that most patients with this condition constantly self-medicate with topical antifungals. Biopsy is usually non-specific and can be misleading. Other than vaginal swab, there is no diagnostic test, and the diagnosis is made on history.

Although a number of factors are associated with an increased tendency to candidiasis (oestrogen-replacement therapy, diabetes, local or systemic corticosteroid treatment, antibiotic therapy and immunosuppression), the majority of women with chronic vulvovaginal candidiasis are otherwise normal. Patients often relate that their female siblings and mother also had a susceptibility to candidiasis. This condition may therefore have a genetic basis. It is exceptional to see it in Asian women.

The first symptoms are often seen around the time a patient first becomes sexually active. The reason for this is unknown. Attempts to relate vulvovaginal candidiasis to various personal and hygiene habits have been inconsistent.

The pathogenesis of chronic vulvovaginal candidiasis is still unknown, but it behaves as though the commensal organism *Candida* is an antigen that causes a maladaptive inflammatory response rather than an infection. If chronic vulvovaginal candidiasis is conceptualised in this way, the condition can be much more easily understood. The exact mechanism is, however, still unknown.

The important role of oestrogen in candidiasis may also explain why patients with a severe problem in the vagina rarely complain of oral symptoms. The vulvovaginal epithelium contains different oestrogen receptors to those in the oral mucosa, and although the presence of oestrogen is essential to this condition, its exact role has not been elucidated. It is known that *Candida* spp. possess an oestrogen receptor but the pathogenesis of how this relates to symptoms is unknown, as is the role of the vaginal microbiome. Research into this during the next few years may explain some of the mysteries of why a commensal organism that is tolerated by most women causes severe symptoms in some.

Almost 95% of cases are caused by *C. albicans*, but other yeasts may be responsible, most often *C. glabrata*. These fungi may be reported as 'non-pathogenic' by some laboratories, and a request for further characterisation should be made if necessary.

Management

If the history is typical, a trial of antifungal treatment should be given. This must be with a daily oral antifungal for at least 1 month. There are two appropriate oral antifungals available: fluconazole and itraconazole. Fluconazole is used at a dose of 50–100 mg/day and itraconazole at a dose of 100 mg/day. Ketoconazole is not used because of risks of hepatic damage over the long treatment periods required.

Both itraconazole and fluconazole have a good safety record and are not usually associated with abnormal liver function tests or frequent side effects. Routine monitoring of liver function tests is usually normal.

A number of side effects occur rarely and include nausea, diarrhoea, allergic reactions, a pustular facial rash, sensory neuropathy, peripheral oedema and, with fluconazole, reversible hair loss. It is very unusual for resistance to be encountered, although it has been described.

It is important to make patients aware that both antifungals may potentially interact with many other drugs including fexofenadine hydrochloride, an antihistamine available over the counter, and statins, which are contraindicated with oral azole antifungal drugs. The interaction with statins is particularly serious and may result in rhabdomyolysis.

Treatment must be prolonged, and the length of time will vary from patient to patient. A useful rule of thumb is to continue daily treatment until the patient is totally asymptomatic. Physical examination is unreliable, and persistent erythema of the inter-labial sulcus is common even when patients have recovered symptomatically. Typically, this takes 3 months, but some patients take much longer to recover, some as long as 6–12 months. At this point, the dose is gradually reduced to the lowest level that will control symptoms over the next 6 months. Again, this varies from patient to patient, and a few are not able to reduce their medication at all without recurrence of symptoms. We find that maintenance doses vary from 100 mg/day in some patients to the occasional 50 mg dose for return of symptoms. The majority do well on 50 mg of fluconazole twice a week. The half-lives of these drugs are such that, for maintenance, intermittent dosing is often effective, although we have found this to be less so during the initial induction phase.

Published reports of the use of oral azole antifungals often recommend 150 mg once a week. Our personal experience with this has been that it does not appear to be as effective as daily dosing in the induction phase. However, there have been no side-by-side trials to establish an evidence-based treatment regimen.

Once patients are on a low maintenance dose, they need to be made aware that a course of antibiotics may result in a relapse and that they should take their medication daily for a week during and after any such course. Any flares of their condition are again treated with an increased dose until symptoms have settled.

Some patients do appear to require higher rather than lower doses over time, and this may be due to a slow increase in the minimum inhibitory concentration of the drug, or individual variations in metabolism and absorption. If this happens, ask about other medications your patient is taking as they may interfere with absorption. Patients with any disease that causes malabsorption may not absorb these medications well.

Once a remission of at least 6 months has been achieved, patients may attempt to stop their treatment; however, many relapse and should be given permission to restart immediately and to titrate their dose to a level that keeps them symptom free. The situation is no different from the use of long-term antiviral medication in the management of recurrent genital herpes, although it is much less well publicised and understood.

It is important to reduce environmental or pharmaceutical influences that may make treatment of candidiasis less effective and increase the recurrence rate. Reducing heat, sweat and friction, improving any medical condition that calls for long-term use of antibiotics (asthma, acne, recurrent urinary tract infections and recurrent tonsillitis) and managing bowel disorders so that faecal soiling is less of a problem are just some of the wider medical issues that should be considered.

The role of oestrogen in this condition means that a symptomatic vulvovaginal problem in pre-menarchal girls and post-menopausal women who are not on oestrogen-replacement therapy is very unlikely to be candidiasis. During pregnancy, symptoms frequently and counterintuitively improve in most sufferers. Although the use of high-oestrogen oral contraceptive pills may be associated with candidiasis, cessation of the pill does not usually improve it. Low-oestrogen oral contraceptive pills are rarely implicated.

At menopause, this condition remits, but it may take up to a year after the last menstrual period for all symptoms to cease. In non-diabetic, healthy, post-menopausal women, vulvovaginal candidiasis is usually associated with systemic or vaginal oestrogen. Chronic candidiasis in this group is usually controllable within 1 month of oral azole treatment if all oestrogen is stopped during this time.

In patients who are unable to cease oestrogen supplements, a twice-weekly dose of oral antifungal medication usually keeps symptoms under control, once symptoms are controlled.

In patients where an atypical *Candida* sp. is isolated, there are two treatment options: boric acid vaginal suppositories (dose 600 mg) or the oral azole voriconazole. The latter has significant toxicities not shared by fluconazole and itraconazole. The same principles of management apply, with daily treatment until symptomatic remission is achieved and then regular long-term maintenance therapy.

It must be stressed that the finding of an atypical *Candida* sp. does not always imply clinical disease in the vagina. An atypical *Candida* isolate should be assumed not to be relevant until all other aetiological options have been exhausted.

Hormone-Replacement Therapy (HRT)-Associated Vulvovaginal Candidiasis

It is important to remember that although healthy post-menopausal women do not suffer from vaginal candidiasis, the situation can change significantly if they begin HRT. However, there may be a lag of up to 5 years of treatment before this occurs.

Patients on HRT may develop candidiasis for the first time, but more often they are patients who have had relatively frequent attacks of acute candidiasis pre-menopause.

Patients who have HRT-related candidiasis require cessation of HRT and treatment with oral antifungal agents until symptoms have resolved (usually 4–6 weeks of daily treatment).

Once a remission of signs and symptoms has been achieved, permanent cessation of HRT is the ideal advice. If HRT is essential, it should be at the lowest possible dose. Maintenance doses of antifungals are often required to prevent relapse. Our usual recommendation is fluconazole 50 mg twice a week.

Diabetes and Vulvovaginal Candidiasis

Diabetes is known to be a risk factor for vulvovaginal candidiasis in pre- and post-menopausal women. The aetiology is associated with glucose load and glycosuria.

The hypoglycaemic agents of the group of sodium–glucose co-transporter-2 (SGLT2) inhibitors are associated with an increased risk of candidiasis in type 2 diabetics, via an increase in glycosuria. Although this can be managed with antifungal agents, there are times when the drug has to be ceased.

Post-menopausal women who are not on HRT but are diabetic may suffer from chronic vulvovaginal candidiasis requiring long-term prophylaxis with an oral azole medication.

The pathogenesis of chronic vulvovaginal candidiasis in these patients is likely to be different from the otherwise healthy group who suffer from it, but is as yet unknown.

Oestrogen-Hypersensitivity Vulvovaginitis

Oestrogen-hypersensitivity vulvovaginitis is a very rare condition that produces a strikingly cyclical vulvovaginitis, thereby mimicking chronic vulvovaginitis candidiasis. Patients suffer from vulvovaginitis throughout the menstrual cycle, with a pre-menstrual exacerbation.

Both endogenous oestrogen and progesterone are recognised as rare causes of cyclical rashes on extra-genital skin. Some women who have cyclical vulval symptoms suffer from this sort of hypersensitivity. The vulval skin and vagina contain oestrogen but not progesterone receptors, and for this reason, the culprit in the vagina is usually oestrogen.

History Taking

Patients often give a history that is very similar to chronic vulvovaginal candidiasis; however, they have had consistently negative swabs and no response to antifungal therapy. They tend to be refractory to topical steroid treatment.

Investigation

There is no commercially available diagnostic test, and diagnosis relies on good history taking and a trial of oral antifungal therapy to rule out chronic candidiasis. In an experimental setting, patients do have positive intradermal tests to oestrogen.

Management

Many patients with this condition are intolerant of the combined oral contraceptive pill. Menstrual suppression with progestogens such as cyproterone acetate has been the most successful therapy to date. Successful treatment with tamoxifen has been described; however, it does have potential side effects. Raloxifene may prove to be a useful agent.

If this rare condition is suspected, the patient should be referred to a specialist with an interest in vulval disease. The use of hormones to suppress the menstrual cycle is best supervised by a gynaecologist.

Extra-Mammary Paget's Disease

Extra-mammary Paget's disease is a very rare condition but an important one, as it is easily mistaken for dermatitis or psoriasis.

Presentation

The presentation is with an eczematous erythematous bilateral or unilateral eruption, which can occur on the vulva or perianal area or both. The erythematous base may have a white, flaky surface that has been likened to icing sugar. With time, the area becomes raw and weeps.

The eruption is usually itchy and sometimes sore. There is no response to topical cortico-steroid treatment.

The typical patient is post-menopausal.

Investigation

Biopsy is essential for diagnosis. The literature states that up to 20% of patients have an under-lying adenocarcinoma, and another 30% have an adenocarcinoma at another location.

Management

Patients with this condition should be referred to a gynaecological oncologist.

Common Pitfalls in the Therapy of Red Scaly Rashes on the Vulva

Prolonged Use of Vaginal Azoles

Intra-vaginal azoles are effective treatments for acute candidiasis but are usually not conve-nient or effective for longer-term use in chronic candidiasis. Prolonged or recurrent use may cause irritancy. If one course of a standard vaginal antifungal does not bring lasting symp-tomatic relief, further courses of similar drugs should not be used, and the original diagnosis should be reviewed. In confirmed cases of chronic candidiasis due to *C. albicans* where long-term vaginal therapy is the only option, we recommend vaginal nystatin, 100,000 U per 5 g dose.

Vulval Application of Topical Antifungals

Candidiasis is usually an infection of the vaginal mucosa only, and the external vulval symp-toms are caused by hypersensitivity to this infection. External symptoms should therefore be controlled with a low-potency steroid ointment. Applying topical antifungals to vulval skin is not only ineffective but may worsen this irritant dermatitis.

Vaginal Swabs

It is essential to understand that a vaginal swab cannot reliably exclude candidiasis. The use of a vaginal speculum to collect the swab is unnecessary. Patients can do their own vaginal swab when they are symptomatic. This eliminates the problem of urgent appointments simply for specimen collection. Nevertheless, the history is more important than the swab in making a diagnosis of chronic vulvovaginal candidiasis. A history of positive swabs in the past is important.

Use of Topical Oestrogen

The use of topical oestrogen for 'dryness' of the vulva may be useless in pre-menopausal women with regular periods. These women are already very adequately oestrogenised, and their sensation of dryness usually relates to some form of dermatitis, as the latter usually produces a dry, flaky skin surface.

Prolonged Use of Potent Topical Corticosteroids

There are very few situations where long-term use of potent topical corticosteroids is required to control symptoms of any vulval dermatosis other than lichen sclerosus and lichen planus (see Chapters 4 and 5).

Although they are appropriate and useful to bring initial symptoms under control, if you find that your patient is unable to reduce to a weaker preparation, it is time to review the diagnosis, question compliance to environmental modification, rule out infection and allergy, and consider corticosteroid-induced dermatitis. Any unilateral or very recalcitrant rash should be biopsied to rule out extra-mammary Paget's disease.

Further Reading

Fischer, G. (2012). Chronic vulvovaginal candidiasis: what we know and what we have yet to learn. *Australasian Journal of Dermatology*, **53**, 247–54.

Fischer, G. and Bradford, J. (2011). Persistent vaginitis. *British Medical Journal*, **343**, 7314.

Fischer, G. and Bradford, J. (2011). Vulvovaginal candidiasis in postmenopausal women: the role of hormone replacement therapy. *Journal of Lower Genital Tract Disease*, **15**, 263–7.

Fischer, G. O. (1996). The commonest causes of symptomatic vulval disease: a dermatologist's perspective. *Australasian Journal of Dermatology*, **37**, 12–18.

Fischer, G. O., Ayer, B., Frankum, B. and Spurrett, B. (2000). Vulvitis attributed to estrogen hypersensitivity: report of 11 cases. *Journal of Reproductive Medicine*, **45**, 493–7.

Fischer, G. O., Spurrett, B. and Fischer, A. (1995). The chronically symptomatic vulva: aetiology and management. *British Journal of Obstetrics and Gynaecology*, **102**, 773–9.

Foote, C. A., Brady, S. P., Brady, K. L., Clark, N. S. and Mercurio, M. G. (2014). Vulvar dermatitis from allergy to moist flushable wipes. *Journal of Lower Genital Tract Disease*, **18**, E16–18.

Hong, E., Dixit, S., Fidel, P., Bradford, J. and Fischer, G. (2014). Vulvovaginal candidiasis as a chronic disease: diagnostic criteria and definition. *Journal of Lower Genital Tract Disease*, **18**, 31–8.

Jones, W. R. (1991). Allergy to coitus. *Australian and New Zealand Journal of Obstetrics and Gynaecology*, **31**, 137–41.

Kapila, S., Bradford, J. and Fischer, G. (2012). Vulvar psoriasis in adults and children: a clinical audit of 194 cases and review of the literature. *Journal of Lower Genital Tract Disease*, **16**, 364–71.

O'Gorman, S. M. and Torgerson, R. R. (2013). Allergic contact dermatitis of the vulva. *Dermatitis*, **24**, 64–72.

Smith, S., Hong, E., Fearns, S., Blaszczynski, A. and Fischer, G. (2010). Corticosteroid phobia and other confounders in the treatment of childhood atopic dermatitis explored using parent focus groups. *Australasian Journal of Dermatology*, **51**, 168–174.

Weidinger, S., Ring, J. and Köhn, F. M. (2005). IgE-mediated allergy against human seminal plasma. *Chemical Immunology and Allergy*, **88**, 128–38.

Things That Look White

White or pale-appearing patches on the vulva are uncommon. Most white vulval lesions are lichen sclerosus. However, vulval intra-epithelial neoplasia may also appear white, as well as dermatitis complicated by lichenification or lichen simplex chronicus.

In the past, white patches on the vulva were called 'leukoplakia' and this term is still used from time to time. This is a non-specific descriptive word that should be abandoned in favour of specific diagnostic terms. Because of the potential diagnostic confusion, white lesions on the vulva in adults should be biopsied if possible.

White lesions on the vulva other than lichen sclerosus are unusual and uncommon; however, there are a few that are important differential diagnoses: these include lichen simplex chronicus (lichenified dermatitis), human papillomavirus infection and squamous vulval intra-epithelial neoplasia. Pigment changes such as vitiligo and post-inflammatory hypo-pigmentation can also present as white patches.

Lichen Sclerosus

Lichen sclerosus (Figures 4.1 and 4.2) is an uncommon skin disease that has a predilection for the genital skin and has a female-to-male ratio of 10 : 1. This makes it relatively common in vulval practice, responsible for about 10% of cases.

Although lichen sclerosus may occur on any part of the skin, it is almost always a genital condition. While we will be referring to 'vulval lichen sclerosus' in this chapter, it is essential to remember that perineal and perianal involvement is common as well.

While lichen sclerosus occurs in all age groups, it is most common in peri-menopausal and post-menopausal women, and the mean age of onset is around 55. It can occur in children and in babies. Until recently, it was believed that pre-pubertal lichen sclerosus resolved at puberty, but recent evidence is against this (see Chapter 9).

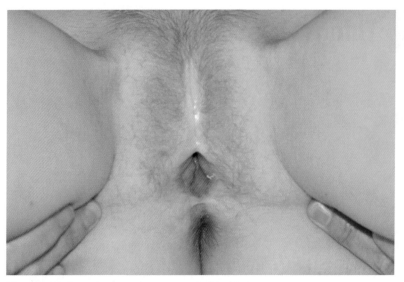

Figure 4.1 Lichen sclerosus with severe anterior labial fusion.

Lichen sclerosus is an important condition to diagnose correctly for two reasons. First, if not treated aggressively, it may significantly scar, shrink and deform the vulva and cause stenosis of the introitus. Secondly, it is linked to squamous cell neoplasia of the vulva including invasive squamous cell carcinoma and high-grade vulval intra-epithelial neoplasia, with the lifetime risk of untreated disease being 2–6%. Both of these complications can be prevented by early intervention, and even with later intervention, cancer and further scarring can be prevented. Therefore, these patients require life-long observation.

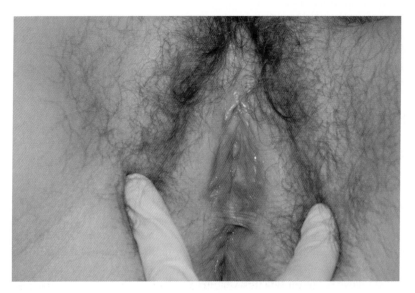

Figure 4.2 Lichen sclerosus with minimal lichenification.

Epidemiology

Vulval lichen sclerosus has a reported prevalence of between 1 in 300 to 1 in 1000 women, and 1 in 900 girls. These figures may well be an underestimate because many cases go unrecognised.

Lichen sclerosus occurs predominantly in peri- and post-menopausal women, although about one-third may occur in women under 50 years. Paediatric lichen sclerosus accounts for 5–15% of all cases.

Extra-genital lesions can be found on any part of the skin but are most common on the neck, buttocks, inner thigh, shoulders and wrists. Extra-genital lichen sclerosus can also occur as multiple small 'confetti' lesions.

In the paediatric setting, lichen sclerosus almost always affects the genital area, with only approximately 6% of these patients having extra-genital involvement.

Aetiology

The true aetiology of lichen sclerosus remains unknown; however, there is a well-documented association with autoimmune disease, particularly Hashimoto's thyroiditis and vitiligo.

Many studies have examined the presence of serum autoantibodies, indicating systemic autoimmune disease such as antinuclear factor, and also antibodies directed at the basement membrane zone of the skin and extracellular matrix protein. The significance of these auto-antibodies is not known, but it would appear that they are not aetiological. It still cannot be said for certain that lichen sclerosus itself is an autoimmune disease.

Should we Test for Associated Diseases?

When patients are diagnosed with lichen sclerosus and start to investigate it on the internet, they invariably discover frightening accounts of associated diseases. This has to be put into perspective.

The following conditions have been linked to lichen sclerosus:

- Autoimmune thyroiditis
- Vitiligo
- Morphoea (localised scleroderma)
- Alopecia areata
- Pernicious anaemia
- Diabetes
- Psoriasis
- Coeliac disease
- Rheumatoid arthritis

Studies claim high rates of autoimmune disease in patients with lichen sclerosus and even higher levels of detection of autoantibodies, but many of these studies were not controlled. A confounding factor is that middle-aged female patients (the main cohort with this condition) have a relatively high rate of autoantibodies.

A recent well-conducted study found that, relative to aged-matched controls, lichen sclerosus patients do suffer from autoimmune disease more often: about 30% as opposed to 10% in the whole population. In addition, about 30% had a positive family history. However, the same study found that there was no significant difference in the rate of autoantibody detection between patients with lichen sclerosus and controls. The two diseases seen most often were thyroid disease and vitiligo.

The majority of patients we encounter with lichen sclerosus are otherwise well with no personal or family history of autoimmune disease. It is not uncommon to find low-titre positive antinuclear factor antibody; however, this is rarely significant enough to warrant further investigation. Thyroid autoantibodies may also be present, and if this is the case, further investigation is warranted. Even in the presence of thyroid autoantibodies, thyroid function is commonly normal.

The question remains as to whether it is best practice to investigate all patients with lichen sclerosus for evidence of autoimmune tendencies. Most patients who have associated autoimmune disease are already diagnosed when we encounter them, but occasionally we do identify patients with thyroid autoantibodies who were unaware that there was a problem.

We recommend only testing for thyroid-stimulating hormone and thyroid autoantibodies. Other non-directed testing is likely to have a very low yield.

Genetic Factors

Lichen sclerosus has been reported to run in families and there have been attempts to find a genetic association. Although no association with the autoimmune-related HLA antigens (HLA A1, B8 and DR3) has been reported, the HLA class II antigen HLA DQ7 has the strongest association with lichen sclerosus.

While these documented HLA associations are of interest, unfortunately there is a lack of significant data to comment conclusively on the strength of these associations.

Presentation

The most common presenting symptom is itch, often of a severe, life- and sleep-disrupting nature. There is sometimes pain as a result of excoriation or fissuring. Distressing clitoral hyperaesthesia may occur, and dyspareunia is very common. However, occasionally lichen sclerosus can be completely asymptomatic, discovered by chance by the patient or by the general practitioner during a Pap test. This is rare but important, as the disease may be advanced at presentation.

The appearance of a well-defined white sclerotic plaque with an atrophic wrinkled surface and areas of purpura and erosion is typical. However, there are many variations. These include:

- Multiple white papules or macules
- Hyperkeratotic lesions
- Plaques limited to small areas such as the tips of the labia minora, the clitoris or the clitoral hood
- Oedema on a background of pallor
- Telangiectasia, purpura or haemorrhagic blistering on a background of pallor
- Fissures or traumatic ulcers
- Erosions
- Lichen sclerosus associated with vulval psoriasis, which appears erythematous
- Brown hyperpigmentation similar to melanosis vulvae, which can supervene

The distribution of lichen sclerosus is also very variable. The classic textbook description is of a figure of eight encircling the vulva, perineum and perianal skin. However, it can affect only the perianal region, clitoris and internal surface of the labia majora, labia minora and vaginal opening (introitus). Lichen sclerosus does not involve the vagina proper (i.e. within the hymen).

A key point in recognising lichen sclerosus, particularly in the late stage, is that the vulval shape is not normal. Virtually all normal women develop labia minora. If these are missing or if the clitoris has shrunk or is buried under scar tissue, this is very suggestive of this condition.

Lichen sclerosus obeys what is called the Koebner phenomenon, which means it localises into areas of friction and trauma. This possibly explains why it is usually most recalcitrant on the perineum and the inner surfaces of the labia minora.

If left untreated, the labia minora eventually become reabsorbed and the clitoris becomes entrapped and buried, revealing an overall atrophic, shiny, white vulva missing normal anatomy. It is very typical for the labia minora to fuse, most commonly posteriorly but also anteriorly. The fusion line is brittle and easily tears during intercourse. Perineal fissuring and tearing is also common. Eventually, the vaginal introitus may become significantly stenosed, with pooling of urine within the vagina, simulating urinary incontinence.

With end-stage disease, epithelial change may be hard to find, and all that is left is gross distortion of the vulva.

Clinical Presentation in Children

A recent study of 70 children with lichen sclerosus showed that the mean age of development of symptoms was 5.0 years (range 1–12 years) and the mean age at diagnosis was 6.7 years (range 3–14 years). Another study of 46 children found the mean age of diagnosis to be 7.8 years with a delay in diagnosis of 1.6 years. Both studies indicate that many children suffer for long periods of time before being diagnosed and treated.

In both studies, the most common presenting symptoms were itching and soreness; however, other symptoms or noted signs at presentation are purpura, dysuria, constipation, genital erosions and extra-genital lesions.

Fewer than 10% of the children studied were asymptomatic and were discovered after biopsy for another reason.

Dysuria and pain with defecation leading to constipation are presentations quite different to those in adults, who normally present with itch and dyspareunia. It is not uncommon for children with lichen sclerosus to be referred to urologists and gastroenterologists. If purpura is present, children with lichen sclerosus may be referred to child protection units.

The appearance in children is the same as in adults, and atrophy and fusion of the labia as well as loss of vulval architecture also occur.

Investigation

Although vulval lichen sclerosus generally has a characteristic clinical appearance, a skin biopsy from the affected site provides diagnostic confirmation and exclusion of alternative diagnoses. A positive biopsy is also helpful in counselling the patient about the important long-term consequences and the need for follow-up, and we recommend it for all patients. It is also useful if the patient changes location or medical practitioners. Treated disease may appear normal, and it is important that there is a clear, histopathological record of the diagnosis.

It should be noted that prior treatment with a topical corticosteroid may render the histological appearances non-specific. However, a biopsy from a white area is usually diagnostic.

In children, a clinical diagnosis is almost always sufficient because of the difficulties of a biopsy, and also because neoplastic transformation has never been reported to occur in children with lichen sclerosus.

The histology is distinctive and uniform across ages and genders. The epidermis is atrophic with hydropic degeneration of basal cells and a homogenous pale zone in the upper dermis. There is a lichenoid infiltrate of mainly mononuclear cells in the dermis.

Differential Diagnosis

The differential diagnosis in adults is lichenification of any sort, extra-mammary Paget's disease, genital warts, non-pigmented seborrhoeic keratosis and vulval intra-epithelial neoplasia.

In children, vulval lichen sclerosus has a characteristic clinical appearance and there is little to consider in the differential diagnosis. Lichenified atopic dermatitis can simulate this condition in adults, but is much less likely to do so in children. Vulval intra-epithelial neoplasia, which may have the appearance of a white plaque, has not been reported in pre-pubertal children. Psoriasis may co-exist, causing diagnostic confusion because of superimposed erythema. Vitiligo lacks the epithelial changes seen in lichen sclerosus, presenting with sharply marginated white macules that fluoresce under ultraviolet light.

Lichen Sclerosus and Associated Malignancy

In adults, vulval lichen sclerosus is associated with vulval squamous cell carcinoma and vulval intra-epithelial neoplasia.

Before it was realised that lichen sclerosus could be adequately treated, there was a significant association with vulval malignancy. About 60% of vulval squamous cell carcinomas had histological evidence of adjacent lichen sclerosus. In adult women with vulval lichen sclerosus, studies had shown a 2–6% risk of developing vulval squamous cell carcinoma.

It should be noted that extra-genital lichen sclerosus is not associated with malignancy.

A previous study suggested that the cohort at risk for squamous cell carcinoma of the vulva had severe hyperkeratotic disease; however, it is possible that there was a selection bias to suboptimally treated patients. Our more recent research shows that patients with relatively mild disease are also at risk.

Where vulval lichen sclerosus is associated with malignancy, the histology is often hyperplastic, may show a subtle form of intra-epithelial neoplasia termed 'differentiated vulval intra-epithelial neoplasia' (see 'Terminology of VIN' below), and may lose its pathognomonic oedematous-hyaline layer.

The appearance of a vulval squamous cell carcinoma can include nodules, persistent fissures, hyperkeratotic plaques, non-healing ulcers and fungating tumours. Any change in an area of lichen sclerosus that does not promptly resolve with topical treatment must be biopsied.

There have been no reports of vulval malignancy associated with childhood lichen sclerosus, but squamous cell carcinoma of the vulva has been reported prior to the age of 40 years in patients with childhood-onset lichen sclerosus.

The association of lichen sclerosus with genital malignancy has very important implications for management. Patients must be aware of the risk, be educated about what to look for and be regularly treated and followed up.

Malignancy After Treatment

It would appear that large groups of patients with adequately treated lichen sclerosus have a vulval squamous cell carcinoma rate much lower than 6%. The suggestion has therefore been made that the risk of malignancy is reduced in uncomplicated genital lichen sclerosus that has been diagnosed and treated appropriately. Our recently published prospective study of lichen sclerosus in 507 adult women compared patients who adhered to treatment and those who did not. It demonstrated that topical corticosteroid treatment kept the skin objectively normal and also resulted in minimal scarring and greatly reduced the risk of cancer. This confirms the findings of our previous retrospective study and the observations of other authors.

We therefore believe that the interests of patients with lichen sclerosus are best served by making every attempt at complete disease suppression and careful surveillance.

Malignant melanoma accounts for 2% of all vulval cancers and in the paediatric setting is considered a rare association with lichen sclerosus. In fact, only six cases of malignant melanoma of the vulva seen in combination with lichen sclerosus in a pre-pubescent child have previously been reported. It is important to bear in mind that melanocytic proliferations associated with the condition have been documented. The significance of this is not known.

Management

Lichen sclerosus in adults is a life-long disease that is unlikely to remit. Most patients are unable to stop treatment without eventual relapse, although this may take many months. It is important when counselling them to make sure they understand that treatment should be assumed to be for life. This news is very difficult for many patients to assimilate and it is important to impress it on them at every visit until you are sure they understand. A comparison to diabetes, which most patients understand is not curable, is useful as an analogy.

In the unusual instances where patients have apparently remitted, they need to be kept under long-term observation, as lichen sclerosus can reactivate after years of dormancy.

Topical Therapy

There are two phases of treatment for lichen sclerosus:

1. Induction of remission.
2. Maintenance treatment.

It is now accepted that potent topical corticosteroid treatment is the gold standard for obtaining remission in vulval lichen sclerosus. The first report of this treatment was published in 1991 using clobetasol propionate 0.05%, an 'ultra-potent' topical corticosteroid. Until that report, it had been considered unthinkable to apply such a strong corticosteroid to genital skin, and treatment regimens with weak topical corticosteroids, testosterone and progesterone were used. As a result, lichen sclerosus was considered very difficult to treat.

Since that first courageous study showed that potent corticosteroid preparations were effective and safe, lichen sclerosus has become one of the easiest vulval conditions to manage, and many further studies with potent and super-potent topical corticosteroid have confirmed this as a safe and highly effective treatment.

Lichen sclerosus is in fact so responsive to topical corticosteroid that failure to improve should be reason to suspect that the diagnosis is wrong, the patient is not using the treatment or there are other factors confounding it, such as allergy or superinfection.

Most of the subsequent studies have also used clobetasol propionate, with more recent studies comparing its efficacy with that of mometasone furoate 0.1%. Our experience has been that, in almost all cases, less potent products will produce results that are just as good. The clinician should first decide if the lesions are more or less hyperkeratotic, and match the potency of the topical steroid to the severity of the skin disease.

The main focus of treatment should not be on the product used but on the end result: attaining and maintaining normal skin. There is no single way to do this, and clinicians can make their own judgement relative to the severity of the patient's disease and their preference for daily or intermittent treatment. It has, however, been our observation that the regimens that work best are used at least three to four times a week. Feedback from our patients is that very intermittent regimens are easily forgotten.

A 2011 Cochrane review was published on the subject of topical corticosteroid treatments for lichen sclerosus. The authors concluded the following:

- The current evidence is limited, and further studies are required to fill in some gaps in knowledge
- Future randomised controlled trials should be commenced to answer questions about the most suitable topical interventions, the potency and duration of topical steroids, and the duration of remission
- A randomised controlled trial to determine if effective treatment reduces the risk of cancer would need at least 984 treated and 984 untreated participants to determine if a treatment can halve this risk, based on a significance level of 0.05 and a power of 0.8

We agree with most of their conclusions, but consider that, in the light of our retrospective and prospective studies, a randomised controlled trial using untreated patients in one arm is now unethical.

Our prospective long-term cohort study of 507 women, comparing compliant with partially compliant patients, has produced compelling evidence that topical corticosteroid treatment is able to prevent not only scarring but also cancer. It has answered this question without the ethical dilemma of how to assign an untreated control group. Our findings in three studies of lichen sclerosus are that, in each group, 30% of patients do not treat themselves adequately. We hope that our research gives us and other clinicians the evidence to persuade them otherwise.

Induction of Remission

The judgement of topical corticosteroid potency is made based on the degree of hyperkeratosis (thickening) of the vulval skin. Although scarring may contribute to severity, it cannot be changed by treatment.

We recommend the following:

- Severely hyperkeratotic disease: super-potent corticosteroid (e.g. clobetasol propionate 0.05% ointment) twice daily until itching has ceased (usually 1–2 weeks) and then daily until review at 6 weeks
- Hyperkeratotic disease: potent corticosteroid (e.g. betamethasone dipropionate 0.05% or mometasone furoate 0.1%) twice daily until itching has ceased and then daily until review at 6 weeks
- Mild disease with only pallor and very little hyperkeratosis: moderate corticosteroid (e.g. triamcinolone acetonide 0.02%, methylprednisolone aceponate 0.1% or aclometasone dipropionate 0.05%) daily until review at 6 weeks

The 6-week review is to check for side effects, the response to treatment and for emotional support as the diagnosis of lichen sclerosus is difficult for most women. At this point, they are usually feeling much better and many assume they are cured. It is important to emphasise that treatment must now be maintained and to explain that the reason for this is to prevent cancer and scarring.

The initial potency of topical corticosteroid is continued until the skin texture and colour has returned to normal. It should be noted that there may be residual hyper- or hypopigmentation (see 'Vitiligo' below). However, the clinical appearance of the surface of the skin usually improves markedly.

Patients are reviewed again 3 months later and then every 6 months for the first 2 years. The potency of the topical corticosteroid is slowly titrated down to a moderate to mild potency for maintenance therapy.

The aim of treatment is the disappearance of abnormal signs as well as the resolution of symptoms. Symptom resolution occurs quickly, but resolution of abnormal signs takes longer. Patients must therefore continue their regular treatment even after symptom resolution. It is important to be guided by objective clinical response. We have found that compliance is best when patients incorporate treatment into their daily routines, and that patients whose compliance is dubious benefit from regular 6-monthly reviews.

The average time to return to normal skin once treatment is commenced is 4–6 months of continuous treatment.

Maintenance Treatment

Regimens for maintenance treatment of lichen sclerosus are much less well researched and as a result less defined than those for initial disease control. Although many reviews and published articles state that the condition does not spontaneously resolve and has to be controlled, there is no consensus on what this long-term control involves. The weakness of most published studies relates to length of follow-up. For almost all publications, the longest period of observation documented is 3 years.

There are two exceptions: a descriptive cohort study from the UK, with a mean length of follow-up of 66 months and a long-term study from France, which was conducted prospectively over 10 years. This latter study of 83 women is the best evidence we have to confirm what most experienced practitioners know: that although topical corticosteroid easily induces remission, it does not cure lichen sclerosus. This study reported an 84% recurrence rate if treatment was ceased. Both these studies suggested that treatment might also change the course of the disease, reducing the risk of cancer and scarring. Our own studies, referred to above, support this conclusion.

The maintenance regimen used in the French and UK studies was intermittent clobetasol propionate once to three times a week, and this is what most other published papers have stated ever since. However, there is no single way to treat lichen sclerosus long term, because differing degrees of severity require different regimes. What is important is maintenance of normal skin texture and colour.

The main potential problems with long-term use of potent topical corticosteroids on the genital area are atrophy, evidenced by fragility and striae, periorificial dermatitis and superinfection with *Candida albicans*. Interestingly, the French and UK studies and another from the UK with a 3-year follow-up period recorded that such side effects were rare when treating lichen sclerosus. This has been our experience as well. In our own studies, side effects were minimal and reversible, and were confined to skin fragility and erythema. The argument that long-term topical corticosteroid use will produce atrophy is therefore not valid in lichen sclerosus.

We recommend that treatment is re-evaluated every 6 months in order to determine the lowest maintenance regimen that will ensure continuing remission. Topical corticosteroid treatment is constantly titrated to the degree of hyperkeratosis. If this relapses, the strength of treatment increases. If atrophy or corticosteroid-induced dermatitis occurs, it is reduced. We have found this method of managing lichen sclerosus patients long term to be successful, safe, inexpensive and outstandingly effective. None of our compliant patients has developed a cancer, and over 95% have had no further disease progression or scarring. Over 90% have complete and sustained symptom control, and of those who are sexually active, over 90% no longer experience dyspareunia.

We strongly discourage regimens that are used on an 'as-needed' basis to control symptoms only. Symptom control in lichen sclerosus is not difficult to achieve, but objective disease suppression should be the target outcome, otherwise the patient is still at risk of complications. It is a common theme among patients who have succumbed to cancer or disease progression as a result of poor compliance with treatment that they had remained asymptomatic.

Our recommended long-term follow-up regimen is as follows:

- Patients are reviewed every 6 months until they have been in a stable remission for 2 years, and then yearly with the proviso that they have an examination by their general practitioner half way through that year and come back earlier if they have any concerns.
- If evidence of relapse occurs on treatment, a more potent corticosteroid is used until this settles.
- If there is evidence of corticosteroid excess, less is used. Corticosteroid excess usually evidences itself with vulval redness and burning or fragility. This reverses quickly once treatment is adjusted.
- Patients should be encouraged not to stop treatment once they are in remission but to continue with the lowest dose of corticosteroid possible to maintain complete objective normality. The psychological impact of a recurrence on a patient who is finally in remission after years of suffering can be devastating. Furthermore, patients who do not comply with treatment have a 50% risk of scarring and a 5% risk of developing malignancy. Each review is an opportunity to remind your patient of the importance and safety of maintenance treatment.

The main outcome measures of treatment are:

- Symptom control: no itch or soreness is expected
- The ability to have intercourse: in post-menopausal women this may also require topical oestrogen to reduce vaginal dryness
- Prevention of scarring, fusion and loss of clitoral substance (a reduction in the labia minora after menopause is common and not problematic but is not always prevented by treatment)
- Prevention of malignancy
- Lack of side effects

Side Effects of Treatment

Side effects are remarkably few. We rarely see corticosteroid-induced atrophy.

We have encountered the following:

- Candidiasis: this is easily controlled with antifungal therapy
- Erythema: this responds rapidly to a reduction in corticosteroid strength
- Stinging from topical therapy: this usually settles as fissures and erosions heal; it is virtually always possible to find a well-tolerated topical corticosteroid

Some patients may have recalcitrant thickened areas that appear non-responsive even to super-potent corticosteroid. These should always be biopsied to rule out malignancy. Such lesions may respond to intra-lesional corticosteroid if they are causing distress.

Newer treatments for very recalcitrant hyperkeratotic lichen sclerosus include intra-lesional platelet-rich plasma. This has been incorrectly termed 'stem-cell treatment' on the internet. Our own experience of this treatment is that it does appear to help some patients, but it is still experimental. There have been no published trials.

In some patients with very hyperkeratotic disease, ablative laser treatment can be a useful adjunct to treatment. However, it is not a substitute for topical therapy.

The most important principle is to maintain observation. This condition is pre-malignant, potentially unpredictable and liable to recur if patients become complacent about its management. It has been argued by some authors that this type of approach is a burden on the health system. However, we argue that lichen sclerosus is not a common disease and that the cost of even one patient with a vulval cancer should be compared with the cost of follow-up of many to ensure that cancer does not occur.

Other Topical Therapies

Topical immunosuppressive agents, such as tacrolimus and pimecrolimus, have been described as potentially playing a role in the treatment of lichen sclerosus in children and adults.

There has been one phase II trial to assess the safety and efficacy of tacrolimus ointment 0.1% for the treatment of lichen sclerosus and the results were released in 2006. Clearance of active lichen sclerosus was reached by 43% of patients at 24 weeks of treatment and partial resolution was reached in a further 34% of patients. The maximal effects of therapy occurred between weeks 10 and 24 of treatment. The authors who recommend topical immunosuppressives state that they are less likely to cause atrophy. However, we have rarely experienced atrophy in our corticosteroid-treated patients, and when it occurs, it invariably improves with a lower dose.

While there were no adverse events during the 18 months of follow-up, the theoretical disadvantage of topical immunosuppressive agents is an increased risk of malignant transformation due to local immunosuppression. This is arguably an important consideration, given the well-described association of vulval lichen sclerosus and malignancy. Squamous cell carcinoma has been reported in adults with lichen sclerosus in association with pimecrolimus and tacrolimus treatment.

At the time of writing, there is insufficient data to recommend topical immunosuppressive agents to treat lichen sclerosus and no justification when topical corticosteroid use is so effective and safe. Topical immunosuppressive agents have no advantage over topical corticosteroids whatsoever. They are more expensive, very likely to sting and burn, and their long-term safety is not established.

Historically, topical testosterone has been used to treat vulval lichen sclerosus. However, there is no longer any role for this, as it is ineffective and may produce androgenisation in girls.

Similarly, topical oestrogen is of no value, other than to reduce hypo-oestrogenic atrophy in sexually active post-menopausal women.

Management in Children and Adolescents

The situation in children is less well documented than in adults. In pre-pubertal children with lichen sclerosus, there is anecdotal evidence that prompt diagnosis and treatment may induce a remission. Children with lichen sclerosus rarely have severely hyperkeratotic disease and therefore the recommendation is to commence treatment with a potent corticosteroid and to manage in the same way as managing an adult.

Historically, it was thought that childhood vulval lichen sclerosus improved or remitted at puberty. This is not correct. Only two studies have examined lichen sclerosus in adolescents who developed it as children and both have cast doubt on this assumption. A study of 12 adolescents with a follow-up duration of up to 10 years supports the conclusion that remission is very unlikely and also suggested that treatment could prevent sequelae. Once children with lichen sclerosus reach puberty, they usually require long-term management just like an adult. It is therefore essential that parents and patients understand that this condition is unlikely to resolve at puberty, and requires long-term follow-up exactly as in adults.

Our group has recently completed a retrospective study of 46 children with lichen sclerosus, again comparing compliant patients with non-compliant ones. We showed that when normal skin is attained and maintained, progression of the disease ceases, and scarring and atrophy do not occur. Scarring that is present prior to treatment, however, does not reverse.

Follow-up of teenagers is difficult because of their embarrassment about examination. In order to avoid this embarrassment, many will assure their parents and doctor that they are asymptomatic, and as a result may be lost to follow-up. A trusting relationship with their doctor prior to puberty is the best way to prevent this.

Lichen Sclerosus and Sexual Abuse in Children

Sexual abuse concerns often arise when children with lichen sclerosus are examined, because of the associated erosions, fissures, purpuric lesions, bleeding and scarring.

There have been numerous reports of patients with the classic presentation of lichen sclerosus undergoing extensive, inappropriate evaluation for sexual abuse. Although the awareness of sexual abuse among health workers has often resulted in more timely referrals by paediatricians for the proper diagnosis of lichen sclerosus, the added emotional trauma to the family is completely unnecessary.

Sexual abuse is common, and many retrospective studies suggest that approximately 20–25% of all females have been abused as children. However, children who have been sexually abused rarely have clinical signs when examined. A diagnosis of lichen sclerosus does not either rule out or prove sexual abuse.

Surgical Therapy

Historically, vulvectomies have been performed in adults for lichen sclerosus, but the disease recurs. This is no longer considered an acceptable method of treatment and is completely

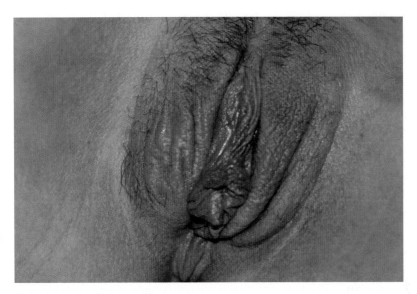

Figure 4.3 Lichenified dermatitis.

contraindicated. Surgery is rarely appropriate therapy in the paediatric population unless significant fusion of the labia has occurred.

Various surgical procedures have been used to treat labial and periclitoral adhesions. Simple division of adhesions gives a very satisfactory result, provided that potent topical steroids are used daily post-operatively until healing is well underway. It is sometimes necessary to apply the post-operative steroid on a dilator. We do not advocate perineoplasty for women with dyspareunia caused by posterior introital fusion. Again, simple division of adhesions works well.

Can Patients with Lichen Sclerosus Resume Normal Sexual Activity?

In most cases, the answer is yes. Physically, particularly in younger women and those in whom the disease was treated before it became too advanced, there is usually no reason why they should not be able to resume a normal sex life.

Women who have had a long history of painful sex have usually developed significant pelvic floor spasm and may need physiotherapy to overcome this (see Chapter 8). Others admit to having developed distaste for intercourse while they were as yet undiagnosed and may need psychological help. There are, of course, many older women who decline any help, because their lack of interest in sex has been legitimised by their disease. Those who want to become sexually active again usually do.

Lichen Simplex Chronicus

Lichen simplex chronicus is also known as lichenified dermatitis (Figure 4.3).

Any skin disease that is chronic and itchy can evolve into a state called 'lichenification'. It is thought to be the way skin reacts to long periods of scratching. In the past, lichen simplex chronicus was thought to be psychological in origin, but this is not generally true.

Underlying conditions that may become lichenified on the vulva include dermatitis, psoriasis and lichen planus (see Chapters 3 and 5). As a result, these predominantly red dermatoses contain patchy areas that are white and have abnormal thickened texture.

Presentation

The clinical appearance shows obvious areas of thickening, excoriation and scale. On the rest of the skin, lichenification usually looks red or brown, but on the vulva it often looks white.

Lichenification does not display the same subtle atrophic, wrinkled surface of lichen sclerosus, and is never bullous or haemorrhagic. It is seen most often on the perineum and perianal area but sometimes is more widespread or, conversely, localised and asymmetrical. It is invariably very itchy.

Patients are often atopic and have dermatitis elsewhere.

Investigation

In most cases, the only way to differentiate lichenification from lichen sclerosus is with a skin biopsy. It is important to differentiate between the two because of long-term prognosis. However, remember: if your clinical impression is lichen sclerosus, particularly if there is scarring or loss of substance, then you are probably correct, no matter what the biopsy shows.

The histology of lichenified dermatitis usually shows evidence of spongiosis and acanthosis (thickening of the epidermis). If your report says 'non-specific', then you may just be dealing with treated lichen sclerosus.

When you read literature on vulval disease, you may encounter the term 'squamous hyperplasia' mentioned in articles on vulval cancer. This is a histopathological term that correlates clinically with lichenification. It may be confusing, however, because it suggests something malignant when what it is describing is completely benign. Squamous hyperplasia is not an indication for surgery.

Human Papillomavirus Infection

Human papillomavirus infection usually presents on genital skin with discrete lesions that are unmistakably genital warts. There is, however, a variant that comes into the differential diagnosis of white lesions, which presents with a hyperkeratotic plaque, very often on the perineum. This can be indistinguishable from lichenified dermatitis, lichen sclerosus and malignancy. Such white plaques should be biopsied, and obviously the treatment for these various entities is very different.

For treatment of genital human papillomavirus infection, see Chapter 7.

Vitiligo

Vitiligo is a relatively common autoimmune disease that results in patchy, very well-defined areas of complete loss of pigment on the skin resulting in striking white decoloration (Figure 4.4). The surface of the skin retains its normal texture, and this is the important clinical feature that differentiates it from lichen sclerosus with which it may, confusingly, co-exist. Vitiligo is asymptomatic and is predominantly a cosmetic issue.

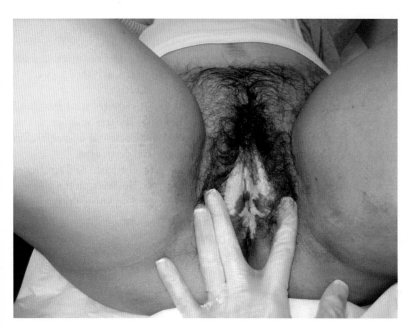

Figure 4.4 Vitiligo.

Presentation

The most common sites for vitiligo are the face, hands, arms and legs; however, it can occur on any site. It usually occurs as multiple lesions but may be localised to one area. This is known as 'segmental vitiligo'. It may also be localised to the vulva.

Vitiligo is harmless. It may occur in association with other autoimmune diseases, particularly thyroiditis. If there is a family history of autoimmune disease or the patient is unwell, further investigation for other autoimmune diseases, particularly thyroid disease, should be carried out. However, most patients are well. Vitiligo on sun-exposed areas presents a risk for severe sun burn because the skin has lost melanin, its natural sun protection. Obviously, this is not an issue on the genital area.

Vitiligo can co-exist with lichen sclerosus. When both lichen sclerosus and vitiligo are found together on the vulva, the clinical presentation may be very confusing.

Investigation

The key to differentiating vulval vitiligo from vulval lichen sclerosus is that there is no textural change. Ultraviolet light is an easy way to confirm the diagnosis, and an inexpensive hand-held device can be purchased online. Vitiligo is brightly fluorescent under ultraviolet light. You need a darkened room to do this.

If there is doubt, a biopsy will diagnose vitiligo. In vitiligo, all melanocytes have disappeared and the inflammatory signs of lichen sclerosus are not present. Therefore, even if lichen sclerosus has been treated and the classic inflammatory signs have resolved, it will still be histologically different to lichen sclerosus.

Management

Vitiligo is difficult to treat. There are many treatments including potent topical cortico-steroids, tacrolimus, calcipotriol and topical psoralens (psoralens are medications that must be exposed to sunlight to become activated and are therefore not practical on the vulva). All treatments are slow to work, requiring many months to become effective.

When vitiligo occurs on the genital area, it is doubtful that it requires treatment, and patients are usually happy to be told that their condition is harmless. The treatments available are likely to be irritating, and prolonged use of potent topical corticosteroid on vulval skin unaffected by lichen sclerosus will result in atrophy and periorificial dermatitis.

When vitiligo and lichen sclerosus occur together on the vulva, corticosteroid treatment of the lichen sclerosus can result in repigmentation of the vitiligo. However, in the absence of lichen sclerosus, potent topical corticosteroids should not be used on vulval vitiligo.

Post-Inflammatory Hypopigmentation

Any inflammatory dermatosis can result in loss of pigment from the skin. This is seen most often in non-Caucasians and in Caucasians with olive skin. It is commonly seen on the perineum after obstetric or surgical repairs.

Presentation

When post-inflammatory pigmentation occurs, the edges are not well defined, and there is often some textural change present because of the underlying dermatosis that caused it.

Unlike vitiligo, there is not a complete loss of melanocytes, and therefore the appearance is of colour attenuation. This means it looks paler than surrounding skin rather than white.

The dermatoses that occur on the vulva that result in loss of pigment include psoriasis, any form of dermatitis and lichen sclerosus.

When this type of colour loss occurs after lichen sclerosus has been treated, it can cause confusion about when to reduce treatment. When treating lichen sclerosus, the key is to observe very carefully for loss of textural change (thickening, atrophy, wrinkling). In some patients, it may take many months for normal colour to return, and in some it never returns to normal.

History Taking

The patient gives a history of a previous dermatosis in the same area, including symptoms of itch.

Management

Post-inflammatory hypopigmentation is harmless and does not specifically require treatment. It usually resolves spontaneously once the underlying dermatosis is treated.

Squamous Vulval Intra-Epithelial Neoplasia

Vulval neoplasia is rare. Vulval intra-epithelial neoplasia (VIN) is the most common form of vulval neoplasia (Figure 4.5) and is seen primarily in patients with lichen sclerosus, or in

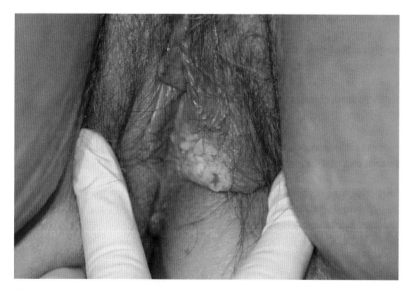

Figure 4.5 Vulval intra-epithelial neoplasia.

conjunction with oncogenic human papillomavirus (HPV) infection, most often with HPV genotypes 16 and 18, which are associated with cancer of the cervix.

Other skin cancers such as basal cell carcinoma, extra-mammary Paget's disease and melanoma can also occur on the vulva, but these are even more uncommon than VIN and are unlikely to appear white as they are rarely hyperkeratotic. The exception is extra-mammary Paget's disease (which can be viewed, in any case, as a non-squamous subset of VIN), which classically is red but may have a white element that looks like 'icing sugar'.

Despite its name, VIN is histopathologically no different from what we call squamous cell carcinoma *in situ* (or more commonly, Bowen's disease) on non-genital sun-exposed skin. Neoplasia has not breached the basement membrane, which in turn means invasive disease has not yet occurred.

On non-genital skin, it is well accepted that *in situ* disease is the precursor of invasive disease. It is not known whether squamous VIN is the precursor of invasive vulval squamous cell carcinoma, and gynaecological oncologists therefore do not regard VIN as a true malignancy.

Dermatologists might disagree with this approach, as they know that Bowen's disease rarely, but definitely, progresses to invasive squamous cell carcinoma on sun-exposed skin, and they see the genital area as part of the skin.

Presentation

The appearance of VIN may be quite different from Bowen's disease. The latter usually presents as red patches, which look very much like eczema. The appearance of VIN is highly variable. Bowen's disease on sun-exposed skin has an excellent prognosis and is usually easily treated with a variety of minimally invasive procedures. In contrast, VIN has a more guarded prognosis and a tendency to recur after the sort of treatment that would be more than adequate for Bowen's disease. This possibly relates to the different carcinogens involved. In sun-exposed skin this is ultraviolet light, whereas on the genital area it is either oncogenic HPV or lichen sclerosus.

The presentation of VIN may be as thickened white or red mucosal patches, hyperpigmented plaques, warty lesions, or persistent erosions or ulcers. The distribution may be single or multifocal, and is usually asymmetrical. Any part of the vulva can be affected, as well as the perianal skin and anus. Unless frank nodules are present, it is often very difficult to tell VIN from invasive squamous cell carcinoma clinically. Only a biopsy will make this differentiation.

Unlike Bowen's disease on extra-genital skin, which is usually asymptomatic, VIN and vulval squamous cell carcinoma can be itchy, particularly when seen on a background of lichen sclerosus.

About half of the patients are asymptomatic at diagnosis, but most symptomatic patients report pruritus. If ulceration occurs, VIN is painful and may bleed. Extra-mammary Paget's disease is characteristically itchy and is often mistaken for dermatitis.

Terminology of VIN

The understanding of VIN has been confused by the previous application of cervical grading systems to the vulva. In the past, a three-grade histopathological staging system of VIN named I, II and III was proposed based on cervical intra-epithelial neoplasia (CIN).

This system was not helpful in describing the actual biology of VIN and was abandoned in favour of a new classification that was published in 2005. This latest classification divides VIN into two types:

- 'Usual' VIN (uVIN): this type is HPV related and is further divided into two subcategories: warty and basaloid.
- 'Differentiated' VIN (dVIN): this type is most often found in association with lichen sclerosus.

Warty VIN is usually HPV related, occurs in younger patients and has a multifocal, warty appearance. It has the lowest potential for invasive carcinoma. Basaloid VIN is more likely to be a single, well-defined lesion, and occurs in older patients.

Differentiated VIN occurs in older patients, usually with lichen sclerosus, and is the most dangerous in terms of the potential to invade and metastasise. This is confusing because when talking about cancer most of us think of differentiated as being less, rather than more, dangerous.

There are a number of names that have been given previously to genital lesions with the same histopathological appearance. They include Bowenoid papulosis and erythroplasia of Queyrat. These are clinical descriptors. Bowenoid papulosis suggests multiple brown warty papules, while erythroplasia of Queyrat suggests red, shiny patches.

You may also read about the term SIL, which stands for squamous intra-epithelial lesion. This plethora of terminology tells us something about how confused this subject is in the medical literature.

The take-home message is that, although controversy exists about prognosis, all types of VIN have the potential to progress to invasive cancer, and older age of the patient and the presence of lichen sclerosus are the factors that make this more likely. From a clinician's perspective, the one term, VIN, is probably all we need for most lesions except for melanoma and extra-mammary Paget's disease.

Epidemiology

Vulval cancer occurs in two settings:

1. Younger women with genital oncogenic HPV infection, most commonly types 16 and 18. Smoking or immunosuppression are frequently associated. It has been shown that HPV immunisation reduces the incidence of carcinoma of the cervix. This may also extend to HPV-associated vulval carcinoma.
2. Older women with hyperkeratotic lichen sclerosus and less commonly lichen planus. These women are not smokers, nor do they have HPV-related disease. They are typically post-menopausal.

There have been few descriptions of VIN before the third decade. Although the two types often occur in different age groups, both can occur at any age.

Any white lesion that is not rapidly responsive to therapy with potent topical cortico-steroid should be biopsied as soon as possible, particularly in any of the settings described above.

Multifocal squamous malignancy involving the cervix, vagina, vulva and anus is not rare, and a careful visual inspection of the entire lower genital tract, including a Pap test, is mandatory.

Investigation

Any lesion suspected of being VIN, including white patches, persistent ulcers, warty lesions, red shiny patches, bleeding lesions, pigmented plaques and papules, should be biopsied immediately.

When taking the biopsy, choose a thick warty area that has not responded to treatment. Biopsies from erosions are often non-specific. If the result of a small punch biopsy gives a non-specific result, refer to a gynaecologist for an excisional biopsy.

A Pap test should be performed, especially in younger women. Any patient with lichen sclerosus should have 6–12-monthly checks for evidence of superimposed VIN, and any non-responsive lesion should be biopsied immediately.

Management

It is beyond the scope of this book to talk in detail about the management of vulval cancer. A number of modalities have been described including:

- Excisional surgery
- Laser surgery
- Photodynamic therapy
- Topical immunomodulators such as imiquimod

Treatment is difficult because of multifocality and the surgical problems associated with oper-ating on the genital area. Most studies report high recurrence rates no matter what modality is used and whether or not surgical margins have been reported as clear of tumour.

Evidence that removal of VIN prevents later squamous cell carcinoma is lacking. Despite this, excisional surgery is currently the gold standard. Some experts have recommended a conservative approach, particularly with multifocal, HPV-related VIN, with only symp-tomatic treatment.

The main risk factors for invasive cancer are:

- Age
- Raised, solitary lesion
- Immunosuppression
- Previous radiotherapy to the genital tract

These patients should always be referred to a gynaecological oncologist for further management. Even if the patient opts for medical therapy, she should first have the opportunity to discuss all options with a clinician experienced in this area.

Further Reading

Bradford, J. and Fischer, G. (2010). Long-term management of vulval lichen sclerosus in adult women. *Australian and New Zealand Journal of Obstetrics and Gynaecology*, **50**, 148–52.

Bradford, J. and Fischer, G. (2013). Surgical division of labial adhesions in vulvar lichen sclerosus and lichen planus. *Journal of Lower Genital Tract Disease*, **50**, 48–50.

Chi, C. C., Kirtschig, G., Baldo, M., *et al.* (2011). Topical interventions for genital lichen sclerosus. *Cochrane Database of Systematic Reviews* (12), CD008240.

Cooper, S. M., Ali, I., Baldo, M. and Wojnarowska, F. (2008). The association of lichen sclerosus and erosive lichen planus of the vulva with autoimmune disease. *Archives of Dermatology*, **144**, 1432–5.

Cooper, S. M., Gao, X-H., Powell, J. J. and Wojnarowska, F. (2004). Does treatment of vulvar lichen sclerosus influence its prognosis? *Archives of Dermatology*, **104**, 702–6.

Dalziel, K. L., Millard, P. R. and Wojnarowska, F. (1991). The treatment of vulval lichen sclerosus with a very potent topical corticosteroid (clobetasol propionate 0.05%) cream. *Br J Dermatol*, **124**, 461–4.

Ellis, E. and Fischer, G. (2015). Prepubertal-onset vulvar lichen sclerosus: the importance of maintenance therapy in long-term outcomes. *Pediatric Dermatology*, **32**, 461–7.

Hengge, U. R., Krause, W., Hofmann, H., *et al.* (2006). Multicentre, phase II trial on the safety and efficacy of topical tacrolimus ointment for the treatment of lichen sclerosus. *British Journal of Dermatology*, **155**, 1021–8.

Jones, R. W., Sadler, L., Grant, S., *et al.* (2004). Clinically identifying women with vulvar lichen sclerosus at increased risk of squamous cell carcinoma: a case control study. *Journal of Reproductive Medicine*, **49**, 808–11.

Lee, A., Bradford, J. and Fischer, G. (2015). Long-term management of vulvar lichen sclerosus. *JAMA Dermatology*, **151**, 1061–7.

Powell, J. and Wojnarowska, F. (2001). Childhood vulval lichen sclerosus: an increasingly common problem. *Journal of the American Academy of Dermatology*, **44**, 803–6.

Renaud-Vilmer, C., Cavalier-Balloy, B., Porcher, R. and Dubertret, L. (2004). Vulvar lichen sclerosus. Effect of long-term topical application of a potent steroid on the course of the disease. *Archives of Dermatology*, **140**, 709–12.

Sideri, M., Jones, R. W., Wilkinson, E. J., *et al.* (2005). Squamous vulvar intraepithelial neoplasia: 2004 modified terminology, ISSVD Vulvar Oncology Subcommittee. *Journal of Reproductive Medicine*, **50**, 807–10.

Sinha, P., Sorinola, O. and Luesley, D. (1999). Lichen sclerosus of the vulva: long term maintenance therapy. *Journal of Reproductive Medicine*, **44**, 621–4.

Smith, S. D. and Fischer, G. O. (2009). Childhood onset vulvar lichen sclerosus does not resolve at puberty: a prospective case series. *Pediatric Dermatology*, **26**, 725–9.

Things That Ulcerate, Blister and Erode

Diseases of the vulva that are primarily erosive or ulcerative are uncommon. Notwithstanding, fissures or excoriations can occasionally complicate almost any dermatological disease of the vulva.

Common conditions such as dermatitis and psoriasis may become eroded by scratching, and allergic contact dermatitis often causes such severe oedema that blistering occurs. Certain conditions, which are not usually ulcerative or bullous, may have rare variants that are. A good example of this is lichen sclerosus (see Chapter 4), which has a bullous variant. All skin cancers may ulcerate, particularly when advanced, and this is also true of vulval cancer.

This chapter focuses on conditions where ulceration or erosion is a characteristic part of the disease.

Lichen Planus

Lichen planus is a rare disease (Figures 5.1 and 5.2). It is very difficult to recognise in general practice, and patients are usually referred to a dermatologist before a diagnosis is made. Despite its rarity, lichen planus always features in texts on vulval disease. This gives the impression that it is more common than it is.

Lichen planus can occur on any part of the skin. In addition to causing vulval disease, it may also cause itchy skin rashes, nail dystrophy, hair loss and oral and other mucosal lesions. The clinical presentation is highly variable.

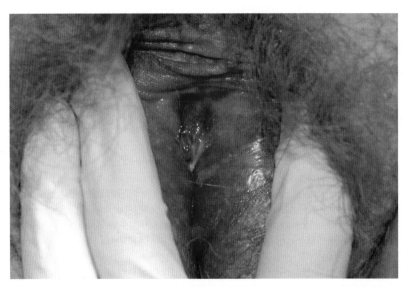

Figure 5.1 Vulvovaginal lichen planus. Note the subtle erosions and heavy vaginal discharge.

The type of lichen planus that involves the vulva and vagina (also known as mucosal lichen planus) is the commonest type of lichen planus that causes vulval disease (Figure 5.1). When lichen planus involves the genital area, it often also involves the oral mucosa, although not invariably. Rarely, it may extend into the oesophagus and anal canal.

The common type of cutaneous lichen planus presenting with itchy violaceous papules with white streaks called Wickham's striae occurs on the vulva (Figure 5.2) but is very uncommon compared with the mucosal type of lichen planus.

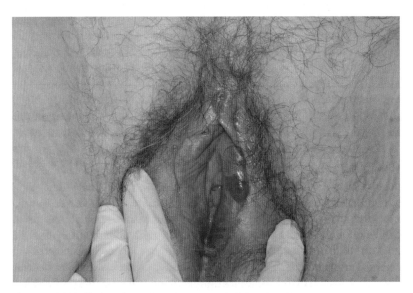

Figure 5.2 Vulval lichen planus. Note the more typical glazed erosions.

It is almost always a disease of adults and is very rare in children and adolescents. The majority of women with vulval lichen planus are middle-aged and beyond.

Presentation

The typical patient with vulval lichen planus is in her 50s and beyond; however, it can occur in women in the second or third decade of life onwards, and in young patients it is a devastating diagnosis. It is exceptionally rare in children.

Patients with vulval lichen planus usually present with pain, dyspareunia and heavy but non-offensive discharge. Itch is not a prominent feature. Dyspareunia is usually severe, and patients have often become completely apareunic. If the anal canal is involved, pain with defecation is characteristic.

When oral disease is also present, patients notice oral soreness and sensitivity as well as tenderness, raw areas and gingivitis.

Aetiology

The pathogenesis of lichen planus is T-cell related, but the exact nature of the disease remains unknown. In a few cases, it is related to hepatitis B and C virus infection, and has been reported to be precipitated by hepatitis B virus vaccination.

Older texts report an anecdotal association with photographic film-developing agents, and oral lichen planus has been associated with amalgam fillings. However, most cases are idiopathic.

Examination

Physical examination is often confusingly non-specific, ranging from non-specific erythema to frank ulceration. The hallmark of lichen planus is erosion of the mucosal surface of the introitus, extending into the vagina and involving the cervix. This presents as glazed erythema, and if one looks closely, the loss of epithelium is evident. Interspersed with this bright erythema you may notice grey patches. This is a classic clinical finding that is very helpful but unfortunately not invariable.

If lichen planus is not diagnosed and treated early, scarring will usually occur. On the vulva, this may involve loss of the labia minora, labial fusion (either anteriorly or posteriorly) and complete obliteration of the clitoris by clitoral hood adhesions. Patients with lichen planus may suffer from recurrent abscess formation because of this scarring, especially on the clitoris. Lichen planus can involve the vagina, and scarring here may result in occlusion or stenosis, making speculum examination impossible.

The distribution of the eruption is usually confined to the labia minora, the sulcus between the majora and minora, the introitus, the perineum and the vagina. However, extension to the perianal area and the anus may occur. As a result, the anal mucosa may also appear brightly erythematous and may also scar and stenose.

Lichen planus is highly treatment resistant, and patients do not respond to weak topical corticosteroids.

Investigation

Lichen planus has a classic histological appearance and is usually reported as being characterised by a predominantly lymphocytic infiltrate obscuring the dermoepidermal junction.

This classic histopathology is easily found in non-genital skin and oral biopsies. Unfortunately, it may be difficult to obtain a diagnostic biopsy from the vulva.

When performing a vulval biopsy to make the diagnosis of lichen planus, never take the sample from an eroded area. If there are grey patches, these are often the most diagnostic.

If your clinical impression is that your patient has lichen planus and your biopsy does not confirm it, it may be necessary to make a clinical diagnosis.

Management

The initial treatment of lichen planus in all cases is with topical and/or oral corticosteroids. Lichen planus is a corticosteroid-responsive condition, but vulval lichen planus must be treated with a potent, not weak, corticosteroid.

The milder forms of vulval lichen planus are able to be controlled by topical steroid use alone, although this needs to be a potent preparation applied daily. We have observed a subset of patients with this disease, usually elderly women, whose condition is confined to the vestibule and who do very well with moderate cortisone ointments applied daily. Even over long periods of time running into years, this is effective and without side effects.

However, the more severe cases of lichen planus often require much more aggressive treatment, including oral prednisone. Because lichen planus requires strong topical and sometimes oral corticosteroids, it is important to introduce a steroid-sparing agent as soon as possible because of the potential for side effects.

Steroid-sparing agents that are available include:

- Topical tacrolimus
- Oral retinoids
- Oral weekly methotrexate
- Oral azathioprine
- Oral mycophenolate

The details of how to use these agents are beyond the scope of this text. If you suspect that your patient has lichen planus, referral to a specialist is highly recommended. We do not recommend treatment of vulvovaginal lichen planus in general practice.

Surgical Treatment

Scarring and stenosis often require correction, but this must only be attempted once medical treatment has stabilised the disease.

Follow-Up

Once lichen planus is diagnosed, it is usually a long-term condition that must be controlled. Our aim is to induce remission with oral and/or topical therapy and to tailor maintenance therapy to suit the individual, minimising this as much as possible.

In our experience, the majority of patients can achieve good control, but it may take up to a year or even longer to achieve this. Not all patients are able to achieve painless intercourse, and a high degree of motivation is required.

Lichen planus is often a devastating and life-changing event for patients, necessitating a huge adjustment in lifestyle including daily medication, some of which involves significant risk and loss of sexual enjoyment and activity. The impact on the patient should never be underestimated.

Table 5.1 Differentiating lichen sclerosus and lichen planus

	Lichen planus	Lichen sclerosus
Anatomical involvement	Vulva and/or vagina	Vulva only; never involves vagina
Erosive condition	Yes, primarily erosion of the mucosal surface of the introitus	Not primarily; however, may split or ulcerate as a complication of the disease
Appearance	Red and erythematous with patches of grey	White; redness only seen with superimposed psoriasis, candidiasis or corticosteroid-induced dermatitis
Childhood	Extremely rare	Occurs in children
Association with vulval cancer	Anecdotally associated with cancer, but association controversial	Association well documented
Treatment	Highly treatment resistant	Responds readily to treatment

Differential Diagnosis

Both lichen planus and lichen sclerosus are scarring conditions where loss of vulval architecture is typical. There are, however, important differences (see Table 5.1).

Other differential diagnoses include:

- Graft-versus-host disease
- Any autoimmune bullous disease, but particularly mucosal pemphigoid and bullous pemphigus
- Desquamative inflammatory vulvovaginitis
- Fixed drug eruption of the vulva

These, and others, are described below.

Graft-versus-Host Disease

This is the condition that most closely mimics vulval lichen planus. Patients with known chronic graft-versus-host disease not uncommonly experience mucosal involvement indistinguishable from lichen planus. Treatment is very similar.

Graft-versus-host disease occurs in 20–30% of stem-cell transplant recipients and is largely a skin disease. Chronic graft-versus-host disease often occurs in the mouth but tends to be overlooked in the vagina, where it may cause significant scarring and make intercourse impossible. It is often asymptomatic until intercourse is attempted for the first time (often many months post-transplantation).

Even when vaginal graft-versus-host disease is symptomatic, patients are often told that they have 'thrush' or a similar minor complaint. It is therefore essential that all female stem-cell transplant recipients are examined at 3–6 months after their transplant, even if asymptomatic.

Only appropriately experienced specialists, in close conjunction with the treating haematologist, should manage these patients.

Desquamative Inflammatory Vulvovaginitis (non-infective chronic vulvovaginitis)

Desquamative inflammatory vulvovaginitis (DIV) (Figure 5.3), also known as non-infective chronic vulvovaginitis, is a relatively recently described and uncommon condition. Its

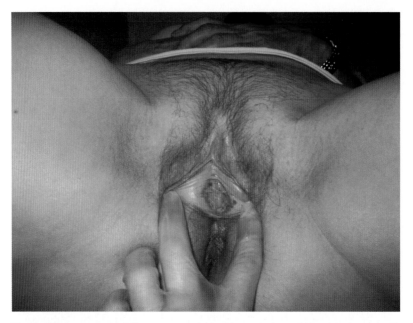

Figure 5.3 Desquamative inflammatory vaginitis with a typical petechial rash in the vaginal introitus.

aetiology remains unknown and controversial. Very little has been written about it. It is not actually an erosive condition, but because it is painful and is very often confused with lichen planus, which may be erosive, it will be discussed here.

We believe that DIV is probably the same entity as Zoon's vulvitis and plasma cell vulvitis. All of these names create confusion, and it would probably be best for international consensus to provide an overarching term.

In practice, although very uncommon, it is still more common than lichen planus.

Desquamative inflammatory vulvovaginitis is essentially a non-infective, non-erosive chronic vulvovaginitis. Like lichen planus, with which it is often confused, it involves the vagina and mucosal surface of the labia minora. However, unlike lichen planus, it does not extend any further, nor does it involve the skin or the oral mucosa, and it does not produce scarring.

Desquamative inflammatory vulvovaginitis was first described 50 years ago. More recently, it was characterised by Professor Jack Sobel, a recognised expert on vaginitis, as a non-infective vulvovaginitis with a typical clinical appearance of erythematous glazed and/or petechial patches on the mucosal surface of the labia minora (Figure 5.3).

Sobel originally described a loss of normal vaginal homeostasis with loss of lactobacilli and predominance of cocci on vaginal cytology. However, the aetiology of this condition has yet to be determined, and studies involving more advanced techniques that might seek to characterise the microbiome of the vagina in patients with this condition have not yet been published.

Sobel established diagnostic criteria based on a case series of 51 patients. These were:

1. Absence of infection, synechiae or stenosis.
2. Purulent exudate.
3. Increased parabasal cells on wet film.

4. Elevated vaginal pH.
5. Gram stain showing relative loss of Gram-positive bacilli and the presence of Gram-positive cocci together with the presence of polymorphonuclear leukocytes.

Desquamative inflammatory vulvovaginitis is not usually a disease of young women and has never been described in a child. The typical patient is in the fourth decade and beyond.

Presentation

The symptoms are usually a combination of soreness, dyspareunia and discharge (occasionally bloody). Itch is not a prominent feature and scarring is never encountered.

The appearance of the vulvovaginitis varies from non-specific confluent dull or glazed erythema, to patchy erythema, to petechiae and petechial patches. A non-offensive, greenish discharge is often but not always present. The rash is never found beyond the labia minora. Although on first inspection the rash may give the impression of being erosive, there is no true breach of the epithelium.

Investigation

Microscopy may reveal polymorphs and loss of lactobacilli, both of which are not specific to this condition. Vaginal cultures do not show any recognised pathogen associated with vaginitis. Group B *Streptococcus* is a frequent isolate, but in this context is not pathogenic. All these findings are by no means invariable.

Published studies such as the one by Sobel cite changes on examination of vaginal wet mounts. The problem for the average practitioner is that most of us possess neither a microscope in our office nor the skills (or time) to interpret wet mounts.

There have been few studies describing the histological features of DIV. Those that exist detail either a non-specific inflammatory response or an interface dermatitis with a heavy mixed inflammatory infiltrate, which obscures the dermoepidermal junction. The pattern is different to that seen in lichen planus. In general, we do not biopsy these patients because of the non-specific nature of the histopathology.

In 2010, we published a case series of 101 patients with DIV. We found that 56% of them had historical triggers, most frequently chronic diarrhoea or antibiotic treatment, while 54% had no significant abnormality on microbiological testing. The previous literature has emphasised the presence of group B *Streptococcus*, which we found in only 13% of cases. Other historical triggers included hormone-replacement therapy and recent gynaecological surgery. We did not perform bed-side microscopy but sought to define diagnostic criteria that could be used in the office of a busy practitioner who did not have the time or skills to use a microscope. These were as follows:

- History: non-cyclical pain, dyspareunia, itch and discharge
- Clinical findings: non-erosive, non-scarring patchy or confluent erythema or petechiae
- Exclusion of other causes of chronic vaginitis
- Drug and irritant causes excluded by trial of elimination
- Microbiology: no pathogens isolated on culture
- Treatment response: prompt improvement with intra-vaginal antibiotic (see below)

The aetiology of this condition remains elusive. Some authors believe it is a mild form of lichen planus. We do not agree with this point of view because:

- Scarring does not occur
- It is never erosive
- It does not involve the external vulval skin
- It responds easily to treatment, without requiring potent corticosteroids

Management

Desquamative inflammatory vulvovaginitis is usually easy to treat. It responds to a number of intra-vaginal antibiotics including clindamycin, mupirocin and metronidazole. We must stress that oral antibiotics are ineffective.

The preparation we use most commonly is 2% clindamycin vaginal cream. Most patients tolerate this; however, in some cases allergy or severe irritation occur. In these patients, metronidazole 0.75% topical preparations may be substituted. Mupirocin 2% is a third option.

Our regimen is:

- 5 g of clindamycin 2% cream inserted intra-vaginally at night daily for 4 weeks plus
- hydrocortisone 1% ointment applied externally twice daily

Almost all patients are asymptomatic and normal to examination by 2–4 weeks of treatment.

Any historical triggers should be modified where possible. If hormone-replacement therapy is implicated, this is ceased at the beginning of the 4 weeks of treatment. If the patient cannot cope without hormone-replacement therapy, it may be restarted after treatment is completed. If the DIV recurs, a decision about the permanent cessation of hormone-replacement therapy will be necessary.

Retreatment or maintenance therapy is often required for DIV. In our study, 95% of patients were symptomatically and objectively improved at initial review. However, 45% of our patients required maintenance therapy. This usually involved application of the antibiotic cream plus hydrocortisone 1% daily externally.

Treatment can be ceased when patients have been asymptomatic for 3 months, but patients should be warned that a relapse might occur. Retreatment invariably results in a rapid response. However, there is a small group of women who had initially presented with a clinical picture of DIV, who subsequently declared themselves as having lichen planus. We conclude from this that DIV may sometimes precede lichen planus. This may have resulted in confusion in the literature, as neither condition is reliably diagnosable by biopsy.

Aphthous Ulceration and Non-Sexually Acquired Genital Ulceration

Aphthous ulceration of the oral mucosa is common, easily recognised and self-limiting. What is not so well known is that aphthae may involve the vulva (Figures 5.4 and 5.5) where they may become a significant problem, not only because they can be very painful but also because the diagnosis can elude clinicians – with unpleasant consequences for patients. The subject of non-sexually acquired genital ulceration, both of the typical recurrent aphthous type and acute form associated with a febrile prodrome, has received scant attention in the medical literature.

Aphthous ulcers are classified as minor or major, the latter being also known as complex aphthosis. Minor aphthous ulcers are small (2–4 mm), superficial and heal quickly within 7–10 days. Major lesions are large (approx. 10 mm), deep, severely painful and can be very slow to heal, sometimes taking many months.

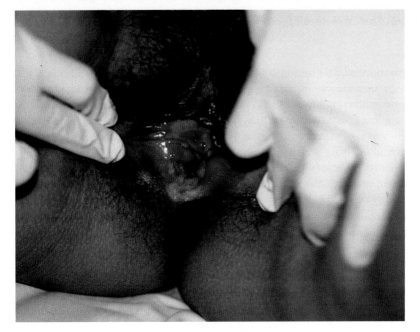

Figure 5.4 Major aphthous ulcer.

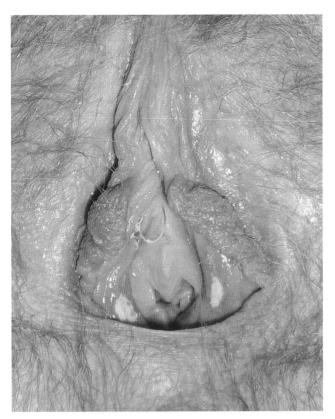

Figure 5.5 Aphthous ulcers showing typical sloughy base.

Aphthous ulceration is by definition a disease without underlying sinister implications. Various deficiencies, for example iron and group B vitamins, have been associated with it, but there is no good epidemiological study to prove this. Oral aphthae have been associated with coeliac disease and cessation of smoking, but this has not been reported with genital aphthae. A tendency to aphthae runs in families. The aetiology is still unknown.

Aphthae are found in all age groups and, although less common in children than adults, do occur before puberty. Patients with genital aphthae frequently have a history of oral aphthae. Recently, genital aphthosis has been renamed non-sexually acquired acute genital ulceration (NSAGU).

Aphthous-like genital ulcers are also found in Behçet's disease and Crohn's disease (see below); however, such patients are otherwise unwell and in most cases demonstrate complex symptomatology. A number of very rare auto-inflammatory diseases such as PFAPA syndrome (periodic fever, aphthous stomatitis, adenitis and pharyngitis) have recently been described; however, these are, like Behçet's disease, complex conditions with features other than oral and genital ulceration.

The sudden onset of severe aphthous ulceration in association with a febrile prodrome has been described, particularly in adolescent girls. It has gone by various names including Sutton's ulcer, Lipschütz ulcer and ulcus vulvae acutum. These ulcers are very painful, alarmingly large and sometimes associated with severe oedema of the labia minora. Some patients have to be catheterised and examined with the aid of nitrous oxide analgesia.

It has been suggested that this very acute form may possibly be a reaction to a viral illness, with the Epstein–Barr virus cited most often; however, many infective agents have been isolated in association with acute attacks of aphthosis. It is therefore assumed to be unlikely to recur. This differs from recurrent idiopathic aphthosis.

Presentation

The onset of the lesion or lesions is sudden and is associated with significant pain and tenderness. In some cases, the pain is so severe that the patient is unable to walk or urinate. This dramatic onset is frightening for the patient and her family. Due to the severe pain, these women often present to hospital emergency departments, where they are frequently subjected to numerous investigations, including for sexually transmissible infections and biopsy under general anaesthetic. The emotional trauma involved usually results in a great deal of anger and resentment from their distraught families when a diagnosis of aphthosis or non-sexually acquired genital ulceration is finally made. This is particularly the case when the patient is a non-sexually active adolescent girl.

Typical aphthous ulcers are round to oval with a yellow, sloughy base and a red rim.

They may be located on any part of the mucosa of the introitus and may be single or multiple. Even when large, they usually heal without scarring.

Where aphthous ulcers are recurrent, the lesions tend to be smaller and less severe, and the patterns of recurrence may vary considerably. Some patients have cyclical recurrences, while others may have constant ulcers for months, with prolonged remissions in between.

Investigation

The most important part of management is initial, accurate diagnosis. If this can be made with confidence, it will save enormous emotional upset for patients with aphthosis. There is very little in the differential diagnosis of such a presentation. Although it is reasonable to rule out herpes simplex virus with a swab for herpes simplex virus PCR, other investigations in the acute stage are unnecessary and traumatic.

Textbooks usually advocate investigating patients for vitamin deficiencies; however, we have never found this to be helpful. Where an adolescent presents with aphthosis associated with fever, Epstein–Barr virus titres are interesting and may explain the aetiology but will not help management.

Management

In the acute stage, the main objective is to relieve pain and facilitate healing. For minor aphthosis, we usually recommend:

- Topical very potent corticosteroid every 2 hours as soon as patients feel the typical pain of an impending attack

For major aphthosis, we recommend the following:

- Oral prednisone 0.5 mg/kg/day as a single morning dose daily until pain has resolved and the ulcer has healed; the prednisone is then withdrawn over the next 4 weeks
- Adequate analgesia
- It often helps for patients to urinate in a warm bath at first

For prevention of recurrent attacks:

- Doxycycline 50–100 mg/day is often very effective
- Nicotine patches may also be useful

Other treatments that have been advocated include:

- Thalidomide
- Colchicine
- Dapsone

We do not recommend the use of colchicine, thalidomide or dapsone in general practice. Dermatologists have expertise in their use.

Any patient with major or recurrent aphthosis should be reviewed by a specialist. Recurrent aphthosis has been associated with Crohn's disease, Behçet's syndrome and two rare conditions: cyclic neutropenia and PFAPA syndrome. If there is anything in the family history to suggest coeliac disease, this should be ruled out.

Crohn's Disease of the Vulva

Crohn's disease may, rarely, involve areas outside the gastrointestinal tract. Many patients who experience vulvitis associated with Crohn's disease are already known to suffer from it (Figure 5.6).

In some cases, the vulval involvement may predate the onset of gastrointestinal tract disease, and cases have been reported where there has been a gap of several years before gastrointestinal tract involvement became manifest, or where it was silent and diagnosed only at colonoscopy.

What is important to remember is that in a patient with known Crohn's disease who presents with vulvitis, extra-gastrointestinal tract Crohn's must be included in the differential diagnosis. It is also important to understand that the gastrointestinal tract disease can be under good control when the vulval disease is not.

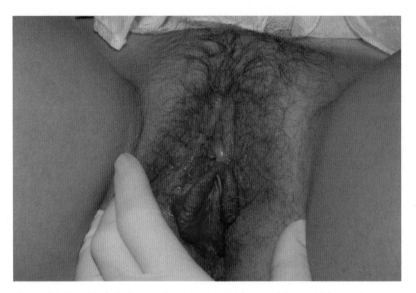

Figure 5.6 Vulval Crohn's disease. This early example shows only bilateral labial oedema.

Presentation

The hallmarks of Crohn's disease of the vulva are:

- Aphthous-like ulceration
- Swelling of the labia majora, which may be unilateral or bilateral
- Fissuring
- Dyspareunia
- Knife-like cuts
- Sinuses
- Perianal erythematous plaques
- Perianal tags

Investigation

The diagnosis is made on biopsy, which shows the typical granulomas found in the gastro-intestinal tract. If the patient is not known to have Crohn's disease already, she should be referred to a gastroenterologist for assessment.

Management

Treatment of vulval Crohn's disease is very challenging. The condition will respond rapidly to oral prednisone; however, for long-term management, our experience has been that it is not possible to withdraw this without relapse. Patients therefore generally require treatment with azathioprine or infliximab. Referral to a specialist is recommended.

Behçet's Disease

Behçet's disease is a multisystem disease found in certain racial groups, particularly in the Middle East, Asia and Japan. It is rare in women outside these groups.

Presentation

Behçet's disease is diagnosed according to criteria, which include oral and genital aphthous ulcers, uveitis or retinal vasculitis, and a variety of inflammatory skin lesions. In addition to these criteria, many other symptoms are reported, including meningoencephalitis, synovitis, myocarditis and glomerulonephritis.

The pathology of this condition is a vasculitis.

Investigation

Although the genital lesions of Behçet's disease may be indistinguishable from minor or major aphthosis, in order to make a diagnosis of Behçet's disease, the patient must have other signs and symptoms, inflammatory bowel disease must be ruled out, and a biopsy that shows vasculitis is desirable.

The majority of patients with genital aphthosis do not have Behçet's disease, and this need not be entertained unless there are other manifestations.

Management

Currently, there is no cure for Behçet's disease. The main goal is to treat and manage the symptoms so that complications do not develop. This involves the use of immunosuppressant medication. If your patient with aphthous-like ulcers has any signs of systemic disease or ocular symptoms, refer to a rheumatologist.

Autoimmune Bullous Diseases of the Vulva

There are two autoimmune bullous diseases that may involve the vulva: bullous pemphigoid, both non-cicatricial and cicatricial, and pemphigus.

Both conditions are very rare. In most cases of pemphigus, it will be obvious that the disease is present elsewhere on the skin and oral mucosa. Cicatricial pemphigoid is often primarily an oral and/or ocular disease, which may also involve the vulva. However, bullous pemphigoid may occur only on the vulva.

Presentation

The hallmark of all these conditions is painful erosions and blisters. It is difficult to differentiate them from each other and from erosive lichen planus without a skin or mucosal biopsy.

Investigation

These conditions usually come into the differential diagnosis of erosive lichen planus, all presenting with vulval erosions. Tissue should always be submitted for histology and also immunofluorescence, which is the diagnostic test.

Management

Treatment is frequently challenging, involving prednisone and immunosuppressive medications. Patients should be referred to a dermatologist.

Cicatricial Pemphigoid

This very rare condition presents with recurrent, painful superficial erosions, which are very slow to heal and do so with scarring. The erosions are usually discrete and few in number. It is a disease of older patients, usually in their mid-60s.

This disease may involve the mouth and the conjunctiva where a similar cicatrising process occurs. In the mouth, it presents with oral erosions of the gingiva, buccal mucosa or palate. It may extend into the oesophagus.

In the genital area, ulceration of the vulva, perianal area and rectal mucosa may occur.

Cicatricial pemphigoid is a very difficult disease to treat, often requiring high-dose prednisone and steroid-sparing agents. Patients should be referred to a dermatologist.

Vulval Bullous Pemphigoid

Bullous pemphigoid is the most common of a group of rare autoimmune bullous dermatoses. It usually occurs in elderly patients, but is well reported in children, in whom it may occur only on the vulva.

In adults, vulval involvement is often part of generalised disease and can easily be inferred from this. Localised bullous pemphigoid does occur, and a specific subtype occurring only on the vulva is well recognised in both adults and children.

Presentation

The presentation is with blisters and erosions, which involve not only the mucosal surface but also the labia and surrounding skin. The blisters are itchy and, once they erode, painful.

Investigation

A diagnosis can be made by careful examination of the skin. The diagnosis is confirmed by a skin biopsy of a blister and surrounding skin. Immunofluorescence is the diagnostic test.

Management

Bullous pemphigoid is not a scarring process and responds readily to oral and potent topical corticosteroids. It is usually a self-limiting condition lasting approximately 2 years. Patients should be referred to a dermatologist.

Pemphigus

This very rare disease usually involves skin and oral mucosa with superficial, painful erosions.

Presentation

The initial presentation is often with oral disease; however, blistering of the skin often follows.

Investigation

Diagnosis requires a skin biopsy submitted for immunofluorescence.

Management

The erosions are very slow to heal and, like cicatricial pemphigoid, the disease is highly treatment resistant, requiring high-dose oral prednisone and steroid-sparing agents. It would be very unusual to find pemphigus involving only the genital area. Patients should be referred to a dermatologist.

Hailey–Hailey Disease (benign familial pemphigus)

Hailey–Hailey disease (also known as benign familial pemphigus) is a rare dominantly inherited disorder. The name benign pemphigus is a misnomer, as this condition is not an immunobullous disease at all. It is an inherited tendency to fragile skin in certain areas of the body. It frequently involves skin folds, and this includes the genital area.

The majority of patients have a positive family history but, as with all genetic conditions, this is not invariable.

Presentation

The appearance on the genital area is of a non-specific erythematous and eroded eruption involving the labia majora. Superinfection with bacteria and herpes simplex virus is a recurrent problem in many patients, and overheating is an exacerbating factor as it increases epidermal fragility.

Investigation

Hailey–Hailey disease has very characteristic histology, which is diagnostic. The epidermal cells appear disjointed and this is often described as a 'dilapidated brick wall' by histopathologists.

Management

Because there is no cure for this genetic condition, treatment involves palliation with anti-infective agents and topical corticosteroids to reduce inflammation. Keeping cool in summer is important. Some patients improve with systemic retinoids. Patients should be referred to a dermatologist.

Vulval Fixed Drug Eruption

A fixed drug eruption is an uncommon adverse event related to many oral medications.

On non-genital skin, a fixed drug eruption is a harmless event, which is more of a nuisance than a danger. However, on the vulva, it may be much more significant and is almost always very difficult to diagnose. The diagnosis may go unrecognised for many years, causing unnecessary suffering.

An *acute* vulval fixed drug eruption is the result of taking drugs that are used intermittently.

A *chronic* vulval fixed drug eruption is the result of daily, long-term medications.

Aetiology

Although many drugs may be implicated in vulval fixed drug eruption, the drug classes that are strongly associated are statins, non-steroidal anti-inflammatory drugs (NSAIDs), COX-2 inhibitors, pseudoephedrine and paracetamol. This means that the offending drug could be an over-the-counter medicine, which the patient may forget to disclose.

Patients who occasionally take analgesics or nasal decongestants often make the connection between their medication and the vulval reaction, but those taking a daily medication frequently do not. Patients who are allergic to ibuprofen and take it for dysmenorrhea often attribute their symptoms to their pads or tampons.

When a patient is on a daily medication, a vulval fixed drug reaction becomes a continuous, chronic one. All therapeutic attempts fail to make an impact and the only treatment that will work is cessation of the drug. Paracetamol is a significant cause in elderly patients who rely on it as an analgesic for arthritis.

The clue to this diagnosis is the peculiar association of recalcitrant vulvitis with an erosive mucositis.

Presentation

In a typical *acute non-genital* fixed drug eruption, the rash occurs minutes to hours after ingesting the offending drug. It is usually an erythematous plaque that may or may not blister. The eruption always occurs on exactly the same place every time, lasts about 2 weeks and usually leaves post-inflammatory hyperpigmentation.

A fixed drug eruption on the vulva does not present in the classic way that it does on non-genital skin. There is usually a bilateral, erythematous vulvitis, which is itchy and eczematous on the labia majora, perineum and perianal area and may extend on to the inner thighs. On the mucosal surface, it usually causes erosions and therefore pain. It does not cause post-inflammatory hyperpigmentation, unlike fixed drug eruption on non-genital skin. This non-specific appearance makes vulval fixed drug eruption very easy to miss.

Unlike acute non-genital fixed drug eruptions, in a chronic vulval fixed drug eruption the link between a daily medication and a chronic vulvitis is usually completely unsuspected.

Investigation

A fixed drug reaction of the skin is a particularly difficult diagnosis for non-dermatologists, as it is rare and slightly bizarre. When it occurs on the vulva, it is even more difficult to diagnose.

Unlike fixed drug eruption on non-genital skin, histology in vulval fixed drug eruption is non-specific.

Vulval fixed drug eruption is a clinical diagnosis that is confirmed when rapid improvement occurs within 2 weeks of stopping the offending drug. Rechallenge is the ultimate diagnostic test.

Management

A drug history including over-the-counter medications, even vitamins, is essential. If vulval fixed drug eruption is suspected, all drugs that can be ceased should be ceased or changed. It takes only 2–4 weeks for the patient to notice an improvement in their symptoms.

It should be remembered that some patients react to more than one drug and that changing the offending drug to a related one may cause the same reaction (e.g. statins may cross-react).

If you are unsure which drug has been implicated, a rechallenge will quickly reproduce the rash. With forgetful, elderly patients on paracetamol, this happens all too often. We usually recommend that they wear a drug-alert bracelet.

Other Ulcerative Vulval Drug Eruptions

Unless a drug causes a fixed drug reaction, it is unusual to see specific ulceration of the vulva from a medication. Some chemotherapeutic agents, such as methotrexate and the antiviral agent foscarnet, are specifically associated with genital ulceration.

The anti-CD20 monoclonal antibody rituximab, used for treatment of B-cell non-Hodgkin's lymphoma, has been associated with severe genital ulceration simulating pyoderma gangrenosum.

Erythema Multiforme (Stevens–Johnson syndrome) and Toxic Epidermal Necrolysis

These two conditions, which are frequently mentioned together, are in fact quite different.

Erythema multiforme is a benign condition of skin and mucosal surfaces, which, although it can cause significant morbidity, is not life threatening. It is usually precipitated by infections with either herpes simplex virus or *Mycoplasma pneumoniae*, although drug eruptions can occasionally produce a similar picture. Very occasionally, it may occur only on the mucosa of the mouth and vagina. It mostly affects young adults but may occur in children or older people.

Toxic epidermal necrolysis is a severe, life-threatening drug eruption where skin erosion is associated with significant multisystem disease. It is invariably a drug eruption, classically from anti-epileptic and sulpha drugs. Mucosal surfaces are always involved, but external skin is often affected as well. However, genital involvement is often overlooked because the patient is systemically so unwell.

Presentation

Erythema multiforme presents with sudden onset of skin lesions, which are classically described as 'target lesions' as they have a round to ovoid appearance with central clearing or blistering. Mucosal surfaces are not always involved, or conversely, they may be the only part of the body involved, but when they are, the presentation is with painful erosions.

The precipitating event is usually either an attack of herpes simplex, which may have been subclinical, or a *Mycoplasma* infection, which may have only evidenced itself with a cough or apparent upper respiratory tract infection. When erythema multiforme is caused by herpes simplex virus, it may be recurrent, occurring after every cold sore.

The diagnosis is usually made clinically, although there is a characteristic biopsy appearance. When vulval erosions are part of a larger clinical picture, a vulval biopsy is not necessary.

Recurrent erythema multiforme of the genital mucosa is usually accompanied by erosive disease in the mouth. The presentation is usually with intermittent and recurrent attacks of simultaneous oral and genital ulceration lasting about 2–3 weeks. The eyes may also be involved. In between attacks, the patient is normal. This is very different from lichen planus, which is chronic, but which it can mimic during an acute attack.

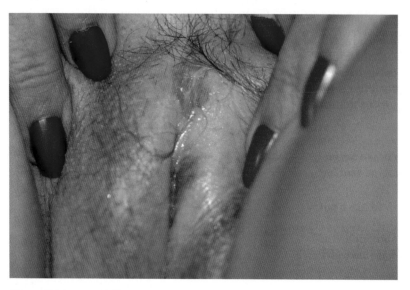

Figure 5.7 Acute genital herpes.

This presentation can be very confusing and normally requires a biopsy to make the diagnosis. The biopsy appearance is characteristic.

Management

The treatment of these conditions remains an area of controversy, but most experts agree that corticosteroids are of value only if started promptly at the onset of symptoms. They are of little value in established disease.

Toxic epidermal necrolysis invariably requires admission to hospital, usually to an intensive care unit.

Diagnosis and treatment of underlying infection that may have precipitated erythema multiforme is essential, but treatment of the rash itself is supportive only. Swabs for herpes simplex virus (see below) and *Mycoplasma* titres should be done, and a macrolide antibiotic as well as an antiviral agent should be commenced. Any drugs that may have been responsible should be ceased.

In both these conditions, vaginal erosion may be severe and may be followed by adhesions, which may occlude the vagina. During the acute attack, intra-vaginal corticosteroid pessaries should be inserted daily, and as the vagina heals, topical steroids should be used with dilators daily to prevent adhesions.

Herpes Simplex

Herpes simplex virus (HSV types 1 and 2) infection is the most common infective condition that causes vulval erosions and ulcerations (Figure 5.7). HSV-2 used to be responsible for most cases of genital herpes, but this is changing because of the tendency for young people to engage in oral sex.

Unlike cold sores, which are usually acquired innocently during childhood, HSV of the vulva is a sexually transmissible infection. It is therefore rarely seen in children. When it does occur in children, however, herpes may not always be sexually acquired, particularly where the child has an underlying skin disorder such as eczema. The occurrence of genital herpes in a child with no predisposing factors does, however, raise the question of child sexual abuse.

Herpes may complicate vulval skin conditions such as lichen planus and lichen sclerosus, particularly when under treatment with a potent topical corticosteroid or during episodes of immunosuppression. Patients may never have had genital herpes before.

Presentation

The first, or primary, attack is always the most severe. Painful blisters are found on any part of the genital and perianal skin and mucosa.

They range in size from about 3 to 10 mm and rapidly erode leaving ulcers. Lesions may extend to the inner thighs and buttocks and may be unilateral. Lesions may be numerous or few in number. Lymphadenopathy is present, and patients may be systemically unwell. Untreated, the attack usually lasts 2 weeks.

Many patients only ever experience one attack of genital herpes, but it may recur at any stage of life with greatly varying frequency. In otherwise healthy patients, the cause of this variation is not known. Patients with human immunodeficiency virus (HIV) disease may experience intractable genital ulceration due to HSV.

Investigation

Diagnosis of HSV is made by viral PCR, sampled by swabbing a new lesion. This technique is very sensitive and differentiates HSV-1 and -2. Biopsy of a blister will also diagnose HSV, but this is usually not necessary.

Serology is not usually helpful in the diagnosis of genital herpes. Positive IgG titres indicate past exposure only and therefore do not help to determine whether the current lesion is due to HSV or not. Rising HSV IgM titres are of value if determined soon enough, but are not routinely required.

Management

Genital herpes is treated with antiviral agents: aciclovir, valaciclovir and famciclovir. The two latter agents have virtually superseded aciclovir because of ease of dosing; however, all are similar in terms of efficacy. The symptoms and duration of acute attacks are reduced by these medications.

For recurrent herpes, all antiviral agents may be used intermittently or continuously, depending on the frequency of attacks. These medications are well tolerated and can be used long term, and they have an excellent safety record.

A diagnosis of genital herpes is emotionally devastating for most women not only because of the knowledge that it is a sexually transmissible infection but because of the long-term, uncertain prognosis.

Although it is not unreasonable to commence antiviral treatment on suspicion of genital herpes, it is equally important to confirm or deny the diagnosis. There are many erosive conditions of the vulva, and not every blistering condition is genital herpes. We have seen many patients suffer for years because of a belief that they have genital herpes based on positive serology alone or simply on clinical impression that has never been confirmed. This can be psychologically distressing. In particular, patients with recurrent aphthosis are often told they have genital herpes, and we have seen patients with this condition not only treated for long periods of time with antivirals without improvement but also under the false impression that they have contracted a sexually transmissible infection.

Other Infections that May Cause Ulceration

In Western countries, persistent vulval ulcers are much more likely to be non-infective than infective. However, the following infections may cause vulval ulceration:

- Syphilis
- Chancroid
- Lymphogranuloma venereum
- Granuloma inguinale
- Leishmaniasis
- Amoebiasis

With the exception of syphilis, all of these conditions are tropical diseases and the patient has a history of living in or travel to an endemic area. Chancroid, lymphogranuloma venereum and granuloma inguinale are usually sexually transmitted. A detailed description is beyond the scope of this book.

Any persistent vulval ulcer must be biopsied in the first instance and further investigations, including culture, PCR and serology, frequently depend on the result of the biopsy. When sending the specimen for histopathology, alert the histopathologist to the possibility of chronic infection. Referral to a sexual health or infectious diseases specialist is recommended.

Traumatic Fissures

Minor tears and splits are common on the vulva, particularly at 6 o'clock on the introitus (Figure 5.8), and usually arise from friction during intercourse or sporting activities, particularly bicycle riding. They heal rapidly in most cases.

Traumatic fissures that are recurrent, frequent and slow to heal may occur in three situations:

1. Where there is an underlying uncontrolled skin condition.
2. Where there is oestrogen deficiency (menopause, lactation).
3. Idiopathic.

It is the idiopathic group that presents the most difficult management problem. This group of patients presents with recurrent, slow-to-heal splits on the mucosal surface of the labia minora following intercourse. The splits are often on the same area each time they occur. These patients have no underlying skin problem and are not oestrogen deficient. As a result, topical oestrogen does not help them. A careful history should be taken, seeking any activities that might cause excessive vulval friction. It is possible for very frequent sexual intercourse to cause vulval or vaginal skin damage, even in the absence of skin disease. Sometimes we need to advise women that they can no longer sustain very frequent intercourse.

Our approach to these patients is to trial topical testosterone, prescribed as testosterone 2% in white soft paraffin. It is initially used every day for 2 weeks and then twice a week only

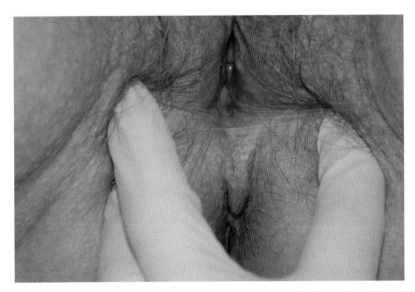

Figure 5.8 Perineal fissures in lichen sclerosus. These are visible only with gentle stretching of the skin.

to the area that splits. If this strategy is unsuccessful, excision of the area that splits recurrently is the next step and frequently ends the problem.

Conclusion: Approach to a Patient with Vulval Ulceration or Erosions

The history must include a sexual and travel history, a search for possible triggers, and any oral or gastrointestinal tract disease.

A very careful examination must be made, and if possible should include a speculum examination of the entire vagina, although this may be difficult because of pain. Look carefully to distinguish between an ulcer, erosion and a fissure. Note whether the rash extends on to the external vulval skin, and if it extends further into the vagina than the introitus. A low vaginal swab should exclude infections.

It is important to remember what is common and what is very rare. This will make it easier to arrive at a working diagnosis. The diagnostic algorithm shown in *Chapter 8* (see Figure 8.2) can be used to help diagnosis.

Further Reading

Bradford, J. and Fischer, G. (2010). Desquamative inflammatory vaginitis: differential diagnosis and alternate diagnostic criteria. *Journal of Lower Genital Tract Disease*, **14**, 306–310.

Bradford, J. and Fischer, G. (2013). Management of vulvovaginal lichen planus: a new approach. *Journal of Lower Genital Tract Disease*, **17**, 28–32.

Bradford, J. and Fischer, G. (2013). Surgical division of labial adhesions in vulvar lichen sclerosus and lichen planus. *Journal of Lower Genital Tract Disease*, **17**, 48–50.

Dixit, S., Bradford, J. and Fischer, G. (2012). Management of non-sexually acquired genital ulceration using oral and topical corticosteroids followed by doxycycline prophylaxis. *Journal of the American Academy of Dermatology*, **68**, 797–802.

Farhi, D., Wending, J., Molinari, E., *et al.* (2009). Non-sexually related acute genital ulcers in 13 pubertal girls. *Archives of Dermatology*, **145** 38–45.

Fischer, G. (2007). Vulvar fixed drug eruption. *Journal of Reproductive Medicine*, **5**, 81–6.

Lehman, J. S., Bruce, A. J., Wetter, D. A., Ferguson, S. B. and Rogers, R. S. 3rd (2010). Reactive nonsexually related acute genital ulcers: review of cases evaluated at Mayo Clinic. *Journal of the American Academy of Dermatology*, **63**, 44–51.

Newbern, E. C., Foxman, B., Leaman, D. and Sobel, J. D. (2002). Desquamative inflammatory vaginitis: an exploratory case–control study. *Annals of Epidemiology*, **12**, 346–52.

Selva-Nayagam P., Fischer G., Hamann I, Sobel, J. and James, C. (2015). Rituximab causing deep ulcerative suppurative vaginitis/pyoderma gangrenosum. *Current Infectious Disease Reports*, **17**, 478.

Simpson, R. C., Littlewood, S. M., Cooper, M. E., *et al.* (2012). Real-life experience of managing vulval erosive lichen planus: a case-based review and UK multicenter case note audit. *British Journal of Dermatology*, **167**, 85–91.

Persistent Vaginitis

Persistent vaginitis is a challenging problem. Women with untreated chronic vaginitis suffer not only because of their symptoms but also due to their fear that they may be harbouring a sexually transmitted infection. Furthermore, once the common infective causes have been eliminated, it can be very difficult make a confident diagnosis, because the available tests are often not diagnostic.

What Is Persistent Vaginitis?

Vaginitis is inflammation of the vaginal epithelium evidenced by erythema, discharge or other changes such as erosions. Infection is the most common cause, but there are less common, non-infective aetiologies. It may occur in isolation or be associated with a dermatosis of the mucosal surface of the labia minora, vulva or perianal skin. Persistent vaginitis is when this symptomatic inflammation either recurs after, or is resistant to, initial treatment.

Most general practice presentations of vaginitis are acute: that is, sudden in onset and of short duration. Most cases are due to acute candidiasis or bacterial vaginosis, diagnosable by vaginal swab, microscopy, culture and pH level, and are promptly treatable with a short course of antifungals or antibiotics. In practice, these patients are often treated empirically. We will not deal in this chapter with the sexually transmitted or tropical infective causes for vaginitis, as the former are covered well in other texts and the latter are usually not a feature of Western medical practice.

Persistent vaginitis is less common and, for the clinician, often perplexing. For the patient, it can be the cause of enormous misery, anxiety, sexual guilt and even relationship breakdown. Historically, it has three patterns: recurring attacks, chronic unremitting symptoms, and symptoms that are chronic but exacerbate at certain times of the menstrual cycle. The main differentiating feature between acute and chronic disease is the duration of symptoms and rapid recurrence after treatment. A previous systematic review has demonstrated that, taken individually, symptoms, signs and tests are poor predictors of the cause of vaginitis.

Table 6.1 Differential diagnosis of persistent vaginitis

Common	Uncommon	Rare	Very rare
Chronic vulvovaginal candidiasis	Desquamative inflammatory vaginitis	Mucosal lichen planus	Crohn's disease
Bacterial vaginosis	Intra-vaginal foreign body (e.g. retained tampon)	Oestrogen-hypersensitivity vaginitis	Immunobullous disease
Contact dermatitis (allergic or contact)	Chronic fixed drug eruption		Graft-versus-host disease
Type 1 hypersensitivity reaction			

Does the Complaint of Persistent Vaginitis Indicate Pathology?

A patient presenting with persistent, symptomatic vaginitis is very likely to have a defined aetiology. Evidence-based medicine in the field of vaginal disease is lacking. There have been no large well-conducted trials, and the publications cited here are observational case series, reviews and expert opinion pieces by experienced clinicians.

Our own differential diagnosis of persistent vaginitis is not long (Table 6.1). The list is based on our published observations and is listed in the order of the prevalence we think may occur in general practice.

Some of the less common conditions that may be unfamiliar to general clinicians include the following:

- Recurrent and chronic vaginal candidiasis (see Chapter 3). The definition of recurrent vulvovaginal candidiasis is four attacks per year; however, there are also patients whose presentation of candidiasis is more indicative of a chronic, continuous process. This is usually obvious on history.
- Recurrent bacterial vaginosis. Although this is usually a single event, in some patients it may recur frequently.
- Type 1 hypersensitivity responses. This can result in itch, burning and swelling, and even anaphylaxis can occur as a result of exposure to latex condoms and seminal fluid.
- Intra-vaginal foreign body such as a retained tampon. This normally presents with a heavy discharge and/or recurrent infection.
- Chronic fixed drug eruption (see Chapter 5).
- Desquamative inflammatory vaginitis (see Chapter 5). This is an uncommon, non-infective, painful vaginitis of unknown aetiology characterised by shiny, erythematous patches and/or petechiae.
- Lichen planus (see Chapter 5). This is a rare skin disease that often involves the oral as well as the vaginal mucosa with very painful erosions, which eventually lead to scarring.
- Oestrogen-hypersensitivity vulvovaginitis (see Chapter 3). This is a rare cyclical vaginitis with a presentation very similar to recurrent candidiasis but not causally associated with *Candida*.
- Crohn's disease (see Chapter 5). This is a rare manifestation of vaginitis.
- Graft-versus-host disease (see Chapter 5). This can present with a picture indistinguishable from vaginal lichen planus.
- Immunobullous diseases (see Chapter 5), particularly mucosal pemphigoid. This can present with vaginitis, but is very rare.

In most patients, chronic persistent vaginitis is not a sign of systemic illness, or indeed infection. It should be noted that, of all of these conditions, only recurrent candidiasis and bacterial vaginosis are causally related to specific micro-organisms. With the exceptions of lichen planus, immunobullous disease and Crohn's disease, which have defined histopathology, none are diagnosable by biopsy.

As these diseases are very different in aetiology, an accurate diagnosis is therefore essential for rational management.

History Taking

A detailed and specific history is essential to making a diagnosis.

The symptoms should be defined as follows:

- Itch, soreness or burning
- Discharge or swelling
- Superficial dyspareunia or skin splitting
- Sudden or insidious onset
- Duration
- Whether continuous or recurrent
- Whether there is a relationship to the menstrual cycle

Historical triggers can be critical to the diagnosis, especially for contact dermatitis, type 1 hypersensitivity reactions, desquamative inflammatory vaginitis and fixed drug eruptions. Vaginal surgery may trigger candidiasis and desquamative inflammatory vaginitis, as can antibiotic use. Events that exacerbate symptoms are also useful, for example the tendency of candidiasis to exacerbate in the pre-menstrual phase of the menstrual cycle.

Ask specifically about the following:

- Medications including over-the-counter medications and whether the vaginitis occurred before they were commenced
- Condoms
- Relationship to contact with semen
- Topically applied substances, lubricants, pessaries and devices such as intrauterine devices
- Presence of oral lesions that might indicate lichen planus
- Previous results of swabs
- Previous response to treatment

Examination

Even though we are discussing vaginitis, there are several diagnoses which may either extend on to the external genital skin (e.g. candidiasis, fixed drug eruptions, lichen planus) or precipitate a reactive external dermatosis (any vaginitis may trigger a reactive genital psoriasis in predisposed individuals).

External examination should be undertaken as follows:

- Inspect the labia minora and majora for erythema, oedema and scale, and note whether there is an accentuation of erythema in the sulcus between them, which may indicate chronic candidiasis. Loss of the labia minora and introital fusion may be associated with lichen planus.

- Look for fissures on the introitus, perineum or perianal skin, often seen in chronic candidiasis.
- Inspect the mucosal surface of the introitus: look for confluent erythema, or the petechial lesions typical of desquamative inflammatory vaginitis.
- On the mucosal surface, look for erosions that might indicate a fixed drug eruption or erosive lichen planus.

On speculum examination (if possible):

- Note whether the inflammation is confluent or patchy: patchy inflammation (especially with petechiae) is more typical of desquamative inflammatory vaginitis or lichen planus.
- Note the type of discharge: recurrent or chronic candidiasis may not produce the 'cheesy' discharge so typical of its acute counterpart. A green discharge may indicate desquamative inflammatory vaginitis.
- Look carefully for erosions, ulcers, adhesions or scarring.
- Make sure there are no foreign bodies.

Investigations and Further Management

A vaginal swab for microscopy, culture (and vaginal or urinary PCR where appropriate) should always be performed to exclude candidiasis, *Trichomonas*, gonorrhoea, *Chlamydia* and bacterial vaginosis, especially if this has not been performed recently. However, if the history and clinical examination are consistent with any of these, a negative swab should not preclude a trial of appropriate medication. Point-of-care vaginal microscopy may be useful for practitioners with the expertise and equipment. Biopsy of an inflamed vaginal mucosa often triggers brisk bleeding, so this should be attempted only by clinicians with the necessary experience. There are no other reliable and valid tests for recurrent or chronic vaginitis, and sometimes trials of therapy are the only option.

If infections and bacterial vaginosis have been excluded, it is usually possible, after the history and examination, to make a short list of likely diagnoses. It may be necessary to rule out chronic vulvovaginal candidiasis by a trial of oral azole therapy (see Chapter 3).

Contact dermatitis and type 1 hypersensitivity are confirmed by resolution of the vaginitis after cessation of the offending item. If the patient has an erosive picture and is taking a drug that has been implicated in vulval fixed drug eruption, the next step is to stop the drug. A rapid improvement will occur within 2 weeks. Rechallenge will confirm the diagnosis in 1 or 2 days.

A non-erosive vaginitis extending only to the labia minora, particularly if patchy or petechial, may represent desquamative inflammatory vaginitis. This is a clinical diagnosis confirmed by exclusion of other causes and by an adequate response to therapy. A 2–4-week trial of intra-vaginal clindamycin 2% cream with hydrocortisone 1% used externally will give an adequate clinical response.

If an erosive picture has not responded to stopping an offending drug (or if there are no suspect drugs), lichen planus or immunobullous disease should be suspected, and referral to a specialist arranged. Indeed, we recommend specialist referral for any perplexing vaginitis case: it is imperative that these women receive timely and effective help to prevent these distressing conditions from causing even more misery.

A vulval biopsy from near (not on) the edge of erosion is indicated to rule out lichen planus. Note that this is highly specific but not sensitive. A negative biopsy in the presence of a strong suspicion of lichen planus warrants a trial of therapy with a potent topical corticosteroid or a short course of oral prednisone at a dose of 0.25 mg/kg/day. A good response is usually seen within 4–6 weeks.

The Patient with a Persistent Vaginal Discharge But No Other Symptoms

This clinical presentation can be one of the most difficult management issues in vulvology. The patient is often very young, and is distressed by what she perceives as an 'abnormal' discharge. She may less commonly describe an offensive vaginal odour, which only she is aware of, or which results from sweating from constantly wearing liners.

Examination and relevant tests are normal, and reassurance is completely useless. Questioning reveals that the discharge has a cyclical variation, is inoffensive and/or of normal consistency. The one proviso is to make sure that the skin of the vulva is also examined. Surface desquamation, which is commonly seen in psoriasis, can be mistaken for vaginal discharge.

It requires great clinical experience to be able to stop further tests and speculative treatments, and tell the patient that her condition is in fact physiological.

Further Reading

Anderson, M. R., Klink, K., Cohrssen, A. (2004). Evaluation of vaginal complaints. *Journal of the American Medical Association*, **291**, 1368–79.

Andreani, S. M., Ratnasingham, K., Dang, H. H., Gravante, G. and Giordano, P. (2010). Crohn's disease of the vulva. *International Journal of Surgery*, **8**, 2–5.

Donders, G. G., Bellen, G. and Mendling, W. (2010). Management of recurrent vulvo-vaginal candidosis as a chronic illness. *Gynecologic and Obstetric Investigation*, **70**, 306–21.

Drummond, C. and Fischer, G. (2009). Vulval fixed drug eruption due to paracetamol. *Australasian Journal of Dermatology*, **50**, 118–20.

Fidel, P. L. Jr., Barousse, M. and Espinosa, T. (2004). An intravaginal live *Candida* challenge in humans leads to new hypotheses for the immunopathogenesis of vulvovaginal candidiasis. *Infection and Immunity*, **72**, 2939–46.

Fischer, G. (2007). Vulvar fixed drug eruption. *Journal of Reproductive Medicine*, **52**, 81–6.

Fischer, G. and Bradford, J. (2010). Desquamative inflammatory vulvovaginitis: differential diagnosis and alternate diagnostic criteria. *Journal of Lower Genital Tract Disease*, **14**, 306–10.

Fischer, G. O., Aye, B., Frankum, B. and Spurrett, B. (2000). Vulvitis attributed to estrogen hypersensitivity: report of 11 cases. *Journal of Reproductive Medicine*, **45**, 493–7.

Jang, N. and Fischer, G. (2008). Treatment of erosive vulvovaginal lichen planus with methotrexate. *Australasian Journal of Dermatology*, **49**, 216–19.

Lara, L. A., De Andrade, J. M. and Mauad, L. M. (2010). Genital manifestation of graft-vs-host disease: a series of case reports. *Journal of Sexual Medicine*, **7**, 3216–25.

McPherson, T. and Cooper, S. (2010). Vulval lichen sclerosus and lichen planus. *Dermatologic Therapy* **23**, 523–32.

Moraes, P. S. and Taketomi, E. A. (2000). Allergic vulvovaginitis. *Annals of Allergy, Asthma and Immunology*, **85**, 253–65.

Murphy, R. and Edwards, L. (2008). Desquamative inflammatory vaginitis: what is it? *Journal of Reproductive Medicine*, **53**, 124–8.

Oduyebo, O. O. and Anorlu, R. (2009). The effects of antimicrobial therapy on bacterial vaginosis in non-pregnant women. *Cochrane Database of Systematic Reviews*, (3), CD006055.

Santegoets, L. A., Helmerhorst, T. J. and van der Meijden, W. I. (2010). A retrospective study of 95 women with a clinical diagnosis of genital lichen planus. *Journal of Lower Genital Tract Disease*, **14**, 323–8.

Shah, A. N., Olah, K. S. and Jackson, R. (2003). Retained foreign bodies in the vagina. *International Journal of Gynecology & Obstetrics*, **81**, 221–2.

Sobel, J. D. (2007). Vulvovaginal candidosis. *Lancet*, **369**, 1961–7.

Sobel, J. D., Wiesenfeld, H. C. and Martens, M. (2004). Maintenance fluconazole therapy for recurrent vulvovaginal candidiasis. *New England Journal of Medicine*, **351**, 76–83.

Lumps – Normal, Benign and Malignant

The vulva is part of the skin; therefore many common lesions found on the skin are also found on the vulva. Some of these lesions can be found anywhere; others are very specific to female genital skin.

This is also true of malignancy: most malignant lesions of the vulva are skin cancers. However, when skin cancer occurs on the vulva, it may have a more serious prognosis than equivalent lesions found on the rest of the skin. Extra-mammary Paget's disease is a specific vulval condition.

Normal Variants

The vulva is one of the most anatomically varied parts of the female body. This is due not just to inherent differences but also to obstetric trauma, obesity, pelvic organ prolapse and sexual intercourse.

Normal variants include:

• Hymenal remnants
• Asymmetrical labia
• Vulval papillomatosis
• Prominent sebaceous glands
• Hyperpigmentation

The hymenal remnants can be very variable in size and appearance, and frequently cause concern. Patients (and sometimes doctors) may mistake them for abnormal lesions.

Vulval architecture is virtually always asymmetrical. As with any other part of the body, some normal vulvas display quite marked asymmetry.

We see more and more young women presenting with concerns about whether their vulvas are 'normal' or not. Usually this relates to the size or asymmetry of the labia minora. In almost every instance, the findings are well within normal limits, but the current media focus on vulval cosmetic surgery, particularly labioplasty, has fuelled many women's anxieties.

Rarely, a young woman will have a very large unilateral hypertrophy that requires surgical reduction. However, in most instances, we try hard to convince the patient that she is in fact normal and does not need cosmetic surgery.

Benign and Malignant Lumps

Other lumps on the vulva can be classified into benign and malignant lesions.

Benign lesions include:

- External genital warts
- Molluscum contagiosum
- Seborrhoeic keratoses
- Skin tags (fibromas)
- Angiokeratomas
- Syringomas
- Fox–Fordyce disease
- Hidradenitis suppurativa
- Sebaceous cysts
- Fibrous polyps
- Hidradenoma papilliferum

Malignant lesions include:

- Vulval intra-epithelial neoplasia (squamous cell carcinoma *in situ*)
- Melanoma
- Extra-mammary Paget's disease
- Basal cell carcinoma

Some of these will be discussed in the following sections.

Warts and Other Lesions

Benign lesions can be divided into infectious lesions:

- External genital warts
- Molluscum contagiosum

and non-infective lesions that may be confused with external genital warts:

- Seborrhoeic keratoses
- Skin tags (fibromas)
- Vulval papillomatosis
- Prominent sebaceous glands
- Fox–Fordyce disease
- Multiple syringomas
- Benign vulval neoplasia (melanocytic naevi, melanosis vulvae and epidermal naevi)
- Lymphangiectases
- Vulval angiokeratomas

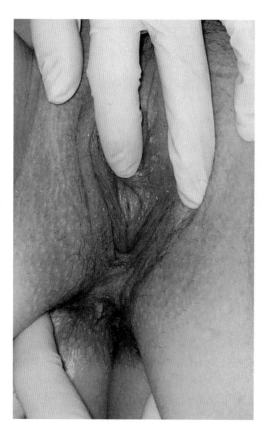

Figure 7.1 Genital warts.

External Genital Warts

Human papillomavirus (HPV) is the most common sexually transmissible infection and is known to cause anogenital warts (Figures 7.1 and 7.2) and also anogenital malignancy. There are over 200 HPV genotypes, but most genital warts are caused by the non-oncogenic types 6 and 11. The risk of a wart being potentially neoplastic is therefore small but not zero.

The prevalence of genital warts in the adult population is about 1–2%, but many more carry HPV DNA on the external genitalia and lower genital tract. Figures range from 10 to 80% and are highly age dependent. As a result of this, people with no obvious lesions can still harbour latent virus in their anogenital epithelium and transmit it to others.

In immune-competent patients, cell-mediated immunity controls latent infection and is responsible for regression of lesions; however, in immune-compromised patients, HPV-related lesions can be persistent and are more likely to be infected with high-risk HPV types, particularly HPV-16, and to progress to neoplasia. This includes organ-transplant patients and patients with human immunodeficiency virus (HIV)/AIDS.

How Are Genital Warts Acquired?

In adults and teenagers, genital warts are considered to be a sexually transmissible infection, spread by skin-to-skin contact during intercourse. The virus is highly transmissible with up to 85% of sexual partners of patients with warts subsequently developing lesions within 6 weeks

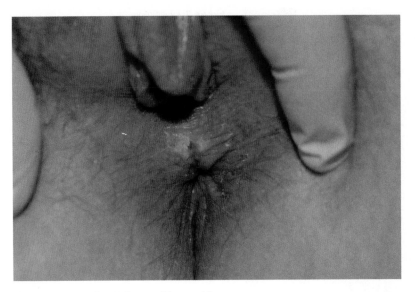

Figure 7.2 Perineal genital warts with central fissure.

to 8 months. The incubation period is not definitely known, but the mean time is around 3 months. It is also not known how long a period of latency may exist where HPV DNA is still present on the genital area after infection, either clinical or subclinical. We simply do not know whether a patient who acquired the virus as a young person can experience a reactivation with clinical warts many years later or whether warts recurring after many years represent a new infection with another HPV type.

The use of condoms does not completely protect against the transmission of genital warts. The reason for this may be that HPV DNA is much more widely distributed on genital skin than the penis, even when there are no obvious lesions present.

It is important to remember that the patient with benign genital warts caused by non-oncogenic HPV genotypes may also harbour other potentially oncogenic types. A diagnosis of benign genital warts does not exclude the possibility of neoplasia in other parts of the lower genital tract and they should be monitored accordingly, particularly if they are immune-suppressed.

In children, however, a sexually transmissible aetiology is highly controversial, and published reports claim that there are many other ways for small children to acquire genital warts. This includes auto-innoculation, innocent transmission from other family members and vertical transmission at birth from an HPV-infected mother. There is very little logic in a medical belief system that immediately attributes genital warts in adults to sexual transmission but denies this in children.

When it comes to genital warts in children, there would seem to be a high degree of denial in the community about how they might have been acquired. The fact is, however, that many retrospective studies show that at least one in five women and one in ten men can recall sexual abuse in childhood, a sobering statistic that should make us all think critically on the subject.

Despite the current media focus on child sexual abuse within institutions, child sexual abuse within the immediate family is a well-kept secret and disclosure is a rare event. With a medical literature that throws so much doubt on the source of genital warts in small children, the best way to manage a child with genital warts becomes a significant dilemma for which there is no straightforward answer.

Presentation

Typical genital warts are raised, papillomatous, often slightly pointed lesions with a rugose surface. The warts are localised predominantly on the vulva, vaginal introitus and perianal skin but can extend into the anal canal. It is not necessary to use colposcopy to see genital warts. They are visible with the naked eye.

In general, genital warts are asymptomatic; however, when traumatised they may split or bleed, causing pain and anxiety.

Warts vary greatly in shape and size. The may be tiny and multiple, cauliflower-shaped or dome-shaped skin-coloured papules or flat-topped papules. The colour is usually skin-coloured to pink to brown and the surface dull rather than shiny. Morphology does not correlate with HPV type. Warts may be very large and numerous, particularly in the perianal area. HPV infection may also present as a fissured, painful perineal plaque that can simulate a malignancy.

The presence of genital warts is not an indication for the use of acetic acid. This stings severely on the vulva, particularly if fissuring is present, and has low specificity for the detection of HPV on skin.

HPV Vaccination

The HPV vaccine targets HPV types 6, 11, 16 and 18. It covers the two most common genotypes of benign external genital warts and the two most common genotypes associated with lower genital tract cancer. New vaccines that immunise against more genotypes will be available in the future.

Vaccination has demonstrated high-level protection against cervical dysplasia for at least 3.5 years after immunisation in adolescents aged 16–23 years, and recent data demonstrates that it has also significantly reduced the incidence of genital warts. It also promises to prevent most cases of cervical carcinoma and vulval intra-epithelial neoplasia. It must be stressed, however, that this vaccine does not stop the need for routine cancer surveillance of the cervix.

Differential Diagnosis

Because HPV is a sexually transmissible infection carrying a great degree of stigma for many patients, it is very important to be able to differentiate external genital warts from other similar lesions. If in doubt, a biopsy will usually provide the answer as warts have a typical histopathological appearance.

The main differential diagnoses are:

- Seborrhoeic keratosis (see below)
- Molluscum contagiosum (see below)
- Vulval intra-epithelial neoplasia (see below)
- Bowenoid papulosis, an unusual variant of external genital warts. In this condition, multiple domed or flat hyperpigmented papules are found on the vulva and perianal area. When biopsied, there is high-grade intra-epithelial neoplasia, similar to vulval intra-epithelial neoplasia.

Management

The appearance of genital warts does not necessarily imply infection from a new partner or infidelity in a long-term relationship. It is important to point out that an episode of genital warts may indicate a reactivation of a latent HPV infection.

There is no way to distinguish between these two situations, and so the clinician must be circumspect, and decide whether it is appropriate to advise the patient to have a full sexually transmissible infection check.

With no treatment, the natural history of genital warts is to regress spontaneously within 1–2 years. Even lesions with histopathological atypia regress. However, in some patients, HPV can be very persistent.

Genital warts are usually not symptomatic and treatment is therefore often cosmetic. Moreover, warts often recur after a single course of treatment, and there is no evidence that any treatment can change the natural history or reduce infectivity. There is no definitive first-line treatment. All treatments aim to remove visible lesions, but this does not guarantee a reduction in infectivity or eradication of HPV DNA from the anogenital skin.

A presentation with genital warts is an ideal opportunity to organise routine gynaeco-logical screening and counselling on safe sex practices, especially for adolescents. A Pap test should always be performed at presentation to rule out significant cervical neoplasia. How-ever, it should be pointed out that the cutaneous HPV infection that caused the warts might also cause a reversible low-grade Pap smear abnormality.

There is no evidence to indicate that treatment of visible warts reduces the risk of cancer development, or the risk of transmission. We therefore point out to patients that observation is an appropriate treatment option.

Because treatment may not change the natural history of genital warts, patients who choose treatment often require a course of therapy rather than a single treatment. In gen-eral, warts located on moist surfaces and/or in intertriginous areas respond better to topical treatment than warts on drier surfaces.

Treatments That Can Be Administered by the Patient

Many patients express a preference for applying treatment themselves. In this situation, make sure that they have been adequately counselled about how to use it and where to apply it. They should be able to contact you if adverse events (usually excessive irritation, swelling and superficial erosions) occur. In all cases, patients should take care not to apply the substances to normal skin. All treatments have a significant failure and recurrence rate, and sometimes a combination of patient-applied treatment combined with in-office treatment can be more effective than either alone.

1. Podophyllotoxin, also called podofilox and podophyllin, has been shown to be safe and effective. Patients may apply podophyllotoxin solution with a cotton swab, or podophyllotoxin gel with a finger, to visible genital warts twice a day for 3 days, followed by 4 days of no therapy. After application, it is allowed to air dry and there is no need to wash it off. This cycle may be repeated for a total of four cycles. The total wart area treated should not exceed $10 \, cm^2$, and the total volume of podophyllotoxin should not exceed 0.5 ml per application. The safety of podophyllotoxin during pregnancy has not been established.

2. Imiquimod 5% cream (Aldara® cream) is a topically active immune enhancer that stimulates production of interferon and other cytokines. Patients should apply

imiquimod cream with a finger at bedtime, three times a week for as long as 16 weeks. The treatment area should be washed with mild soap and water 6–10 hours after the application. This preparation always causes an inflammatory response on treated skin, and care should be taken to avoid excessive inflammation. It therefore may not be appropriate to use imiquimod on introital skin, especially in patients predisposed to atopic skin disease. Many patients will be clear of warts by 8–10 weeks, or even sooner. The safety of imiquimod during pregnancy has not been established.

3. Green tea sinecatechins (polyphenon E ointment). This preparation is approved for use in patients over 18 years of age for external genital and perianal warts. It has been shown to be safe and reasonably effective. It is applied three times daily, leaving a thin layer on the warts. It is not necessary to wash it off.

4. Ingenol mebutate 0.015% gel and fluorouracil 5% cream. Both of these topical therapies used for actinic keratosis treatment have anecdotally been reported to be useful in eradicating genital warts. Where other treatments have failed, in a patient who is very determined to be rid of her genital warts, these treatments are a possibility. Referral to a dermatologist is advised as side effects include severe irritation.

Treatments That Are Administered by the Doctor

1. Cryotherapy with liquid nitrogen. This is suitable only for small lesions. It is important to keep the lesion frozen for 30 seconds, allow the wart to thaw and then repeat.

2. Surgical removal either by tangential scissors excision, tangential shave excision, curettage, or electrosurgery. Surgical removal of warts has an advantage over other treatment modalities in that it renders the patient wart free, usually with a single visit. This is particularly appropriate in cases where the lesions are very numerous and are interfering with function, particularly in the perianal area. In children, a general anaesthetic is usually required.

3. Surgical laser ablation with a CO_2 laser. This has similar application to surgical treatment; however, there is a risk to the operator from aerosolised HPV DNA, and clinicians who do this treatment should be appropriately gowned and gloved.

4. Cidofovir. This is an antiviral drug with activity against a broad spectrum of DNA viruses including HPV. It has been shown to be effective when used topically by the patient as a 1% cream or gel, or intra-lesionally by the doctor. This use is off label and the cost is considerable. There is a growing body of evidence that this treatment is useful for anogenital warts in adults and children, and it may be useful in future.

External Genital Warts in Pregnancy

Genital warts can become much more severe in pregnant women but usually improve after the baby is born. Many experts advocate their removal at this time. HPV-6 and -11 can cause laryngeal papillomatosis among infants, and the route of transmission (transplacental, birth canal or postnatal) is not completely understood. The preventative value of caesarean delivery is unknown; thus, caesarean delivery should not be performed solely to prevent transmission of HPV infection to the newborn.

Cryotherapy is safe in pregnancy; however, topical treatments are contraindicated.

Follow-Up

After visible genital warts have cleared, patients should be cautioned to watch for recurrences, which occur most frequently during the first 3 months.

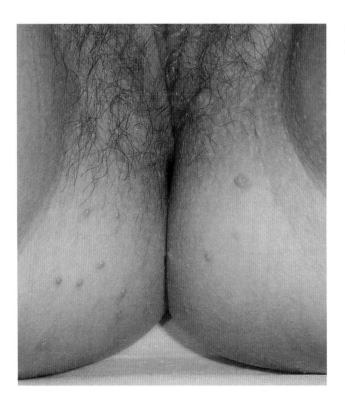

Figure 7.3 Molluscum contagiosum. Note the typical central umbilication.

Treatment of Sex Partners

Examination of sex partners is not necessary for management of genital warts because the role of reinfection is probably minimal. Therefore, treatment to reduce transmission is not necessary. Because treatment of genital warts does not eliminate HPV colonisation, patients should be cautioned that they may still be at risk of wart recurrence.

Psychological Issues

The emotional impact of genital warts is huge. Many patients say they feel 'dirty', and this is usually why they seek treatment for a condition that is asymptomatic. The discovery of warts for a woman in a monogamous relationship may place great stress on the relationship. Because of the unknown incubation period, it is very difficult to be categorical about the source of the warts, and there is often never a satisfactory answer. Couples may need counselling to come to terms with the diagnosis.

Molluscum Contagiosum

Molluscum contagiosum (Figure 7.3) is a viral infection that is very common in children but less so in adults. When it occurs on the vulva in adults, it is usually sexually acquired, but in children it is more common and is usually acquired from swimming pools and siblings with whom they share a bath. Auto-inoculation is also an important method of transmission. In children, genital mollusca are rarely found in isolation without evidence of more widespread infection of other parts of the skin.

There are four genotypes of molluscum contagiosum virus (MCV), and studies show that MCV-1 is the type usually found in children, while MCV-2 is found in adults with sexually transmissible infection.

Presentation

Following an incubation period of 2 weeks to several months, the mollusca are seen as umbilicated flesh-coloured papules of 2–5 mm with a pearly appearance. Giant mollusca can occur on the genital region, and occasionally they may become inflamed and superinfected. Very small lesions often lack typical umbilication.

Mollusca of the genital area are usually asymptomatic, but itch and a secondary dermatitis may occur, particularly in atopic children. Mollusca can be severe in immunosuppressed patients, but in a healthy patient, severe mollusca is not necessarily a sign of any other disease. Some patients are simply more susceptible than others.

Mollusca are self-limiting within 6 months to 2 years in immunocompetent patients but may have a prolonged course in immunosuppressed patients. After they resolve, they are unlikely to recur.

Investigation

Diagnosis is usually made clinically; however, in the genital area, it may occasionally be difficult to differentiate small mollusca without typical umbilication from genital warts.

If there is any doubt, the diagnosis can be confirmed by microscopy performed on material from a lesion obtained by extruding the central core with pressure, a small curette or a simple shave biopsy. Histopathology is highly characteristic.

Management

Treatment of perianal and perigenital mollusca can be difficult in small children but is very easy in adults. Avoidance of baths and swimming pools may reduce auto-inoculation. If pruritus is a problem, topical corticosteroids are helpful; however, topical immunomodulators should be avoided, as both pimecrolimus and tacrolimus have been implicated in the spread of the infection. Unless the lesions are distressing, it may be best to allow them to resolve spontaneously.

Mollusca lesions have a small round core containing viral particles. If this is removed or damaged, the lesions resolve quickly.

Methods that work for removing mollusca include the following:

- Scrape them off gently with a small skin curette
- Squeeze the lesions to remove the core
- Prick with a needle to flick out the core
- Lightly freeze with a cryotherapy unit

Imiquimod (Aldara®) has been recommended as a treatment for mollusca. However, it is expensive, irritating and not completely reliable.

Cantharidin is a topical substance that causes blistering. It can be useful in mollusca in children; however, use on the genital area would be very irritating and is better avoided.

In adults the best course of action is physical removal. In children leaving them to resolve spontaneously while reducing auto-innoculation by substituting showers for baths is usually more appropriate.

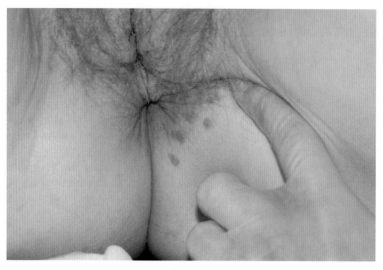

Figure 7.4 Seborrhoeic keratoses.

Seborrhoeic Keratoses

These very common benign skin lesions are common in people over the age of 40 years (Figure 7.4). They can be found on any part of the skin including the vulva. They do not occur in the vagina.

Presentation

Seborrhoeic keratoses have very varied shapes, sizes and colours. They may be flat, raised or pedunculated and often closely resemble warts. Colours range from skin tone to black. They may thus be confused with melanoma. They become more numerous with age.

These lesions are usually not symptomatic but if large may rub on clothing and become irritating. If they are scratched or traumatised, they may suddenly enlarge and darken.

Investigation

The main significance of seborrhoeic keratoses on the vulva is their resemblance to genital warts and sometimes to vulval intra-epithelial neoplasia (VIN; also called squamous cell carcinoma *in situ*). However, they are easily differentiated on biopsy as they have a typical histological appearance.

Dermoscopy is also frequently diagnostic of seborrhoeic keratoses, showing classical follicular plugging. However, it is awkward to perform on the vulva without a set-up that allows a dignified distance between the doctor and patient. This can be achieved by using a dermatoscope attached to a camera.

Management

Treatment of these lesions can be successfully achieved with:

- Cryotherapy
- Light curettage and cautery
- Excision of large lesions

Recurrences may occur but are less common than with external genital warts.

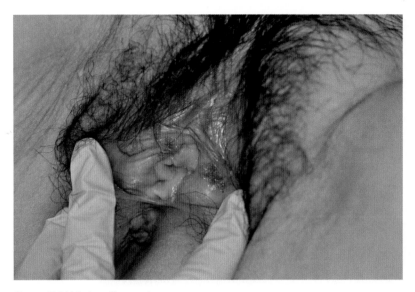

Figure 7.5 Vulval papillomatosis.

Skin Tags (Fibromas)

These harmless lesions are common in the major flexures. They are most often found in the axillae, neck and inguinal folds.

Skin tags usually form in middle age and can occur during pregnancy. The appearance of multiple skin tags in young people is unusual and should prompt a search for signs of tuberous sclerosus, neurofibromatosis or, if perianal, Crohn's disease.

Skin tags are small, soft, pedunculated lesions, flesh coloured to brown in colour. They often accompany seborrhoeic keratoses. The base of the peduncle is rarely wider than 1–2 mm.

Management

There is no medical need to treat skin tags, but many patients request removal because they rub on clothing.

The easiest treatment is scissor amputation at the base of the peduncle. If this is done quickly, no local anaesthetic is required unless they are quite large. Bleeding can be stopped with pressure.

Any destructive method will work: hyfrecation or cryotherapy is also effective.

Vulval Papillomatosis

This is an unusual but important condition because it is very likely to be mistaken for genital warts. Indeed, in the past, the medical literature has suggested that vulval papillomatosis is an HPV-related condition. This is incorrect. Vulval papillomatosis is a normal variant (Figure 7.5).

Presentation

Patients with this condition are found to have multiple small papillae on the mucosal surface of the labia minora in the vestibule.

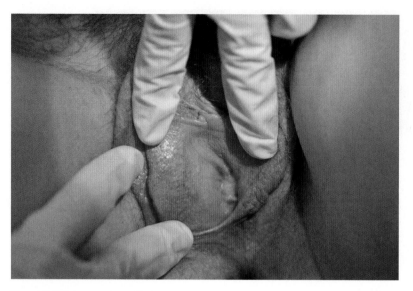

Figure 7.6 Sebaceous hyperplasia.

The lesions are asymptomatic. The main differentiating factor from warts is the uniformity of the papillae, which are flesh coloured with a smooth rounded surface unlike the dull, rough and often pointed shape of genital warts. They are symmetrically distributed.

These lesions are analogous to pearly penile papules found in males.

Investigation

If there is any doubt, a small biopsy will differentiate them from genital warts.

Prominent Sebaceous Glands

The inner surface of the labia minora contains numerous sebaceous glands. This is normal and does not cause any symptoms. Although they are usually imperceptible, in some patients, sebaceous glands are more obvious than in others. When this occurs, they are often described as hyperplastic (Figure 7.6). This term is confusing, because these lesions do not represent a disease state. Hyperplastic sebaceous glands appear as small, discrete, slightly yellowish flat papules. To distinguish this from an abnormality, it is more appropriate to call them prominent sebaceous glands.

When a patient's attention is drawn to her vulva for any other reason, it is quite common for her to become alarmed by the presence of these normal structures.

Management

Strong reassurance that they are not the cause of any vulval symptoms is all that is required.

Fox–Fordyce Disease

This is a benign and very rare condition of unknown aetiology.

The onset of this condition is usually in adolescence to young adulthood; however, there have been cases reported in children.

The pathology of this condition has been described as inflammation of the hair follicle, but the histopathology is essentially non-specific.

Presentation

Multiple 2–4 mm, itchy, dome-shaped papules occur bilaterally on the vulva and pubic area. They often also occur in the axillae and on the areolae. It is therefore said that this represents a disorder of apocrine glands because these are the areas where they are located. The glands are connected to the hair follicle in these areas and secrete an oily fluid, which is different to sweat.

Management

Treatment of Fox–Fordyce disease is difficult. Many strategies and topical therapies have been suggested including topical retinoids, corticosteroids, antibiotics and surgical removal of the affected area.

A recent case report indicated that topical pimecrolimus was of benefit. We have also found topical tacrolimus to be useful.

Multiple Syringomas

Syringomas are benign adnexal tumours, consisting of eccrine sweat glands. They are usually multiple and are found most commonly under the eyes.

Presentation

There is a variant of multiple syringoma that is found on the vulva. It presents with multiple, small, round papules, which are usually flesh coloured but may also be brown or violaceous. The distribution is usually on the labia majora bilaterally. They may be very numerous or few in number.

The onset of these lesions is usually in adolescence or early adult life. Although on other body sites they are not symptomatic and present only a cosmetic problem, on the vulva they may be intractably itchy.

Investigation

The histopathology is characteristic, demonstrating multiple clusters of eccrine glands in the dermis. Biopsy is diagnostic. This helps to differentiate them from Fox–Fordyce disease.

Management

Multiple itchy syringomata on the vulva can be a difficult clinical problem. Topical therapy with anti-inflammatory agents may be ineffective. Topical atropine has been reported to reduce itch; however, definitive management is surgical removal of the skin involved.

Benign Vulval Neoplasia

Naevi and other benign neoplastic lesions may occur on any part of the skin and this includes the vulva. Such lesions are divided into four categories:

- Melanocytic naevi
- Vascular lesions of early and late onset
- Epidermal naevi
- Acquired benign tumours

Melanocytic Naevi

Melanocytic naevi are quite common on the vulva and look no different from similar lesions on any other part of the skin.

Presentation

They present as small, slightly raised or pedunculated pink to brown papules, which may or may not grow hair. They generally appear from childhood until the mid-20s.

Melanocytic naevi evolve slowly with time, gradually regressing with age.

On the vulva, melanocytic naevi rarely cause any morbidity unless they rub on clothes. Patients are often anxious about their potential to become malignant (see 'Melanoma of the vulva' below).

The potential for any given small melanocytic naevus to develop into a malignant melanoma is very small. This is just as true for vulval naevi as for naevi on any other part of the skin and preventative removal is not necessary. The main indication for removal is cosmetic or functional.

Examination

Evaluation of a vulval melanocytic naevus is no different to a naevus elsewhere; however, in practice it is difficult to use a dermatoscope on the vulva for obvious reasons. The use of a dermatoscope with a camera set-up that allows photography of melanocytic lesions is a solution to this problem, but the equipment is expensive.

Photography and simple measurement are a good way to monitor melanocytic lesions. If such lesions have benign features, they can safely be observed. These features are:

- Even colour
- Regular border
- Symmetry
- Lack of itch or bleeding
- Stability (remembering that over several years features may slowly change)

Epidermal Naevi

In general, these lesions are uncommon and even less common on the vulva. They are hamartomas that usually appear in the first few years of life, extend for a few years, and then stabilise and persist throughout life.

There are many different types of epidermal naevi. On the vulva, the usual type is the keratinocytic or verrucous epidermal naevus.

Presentation

The clinical presentation is of a flesh coloured to brown keratotic papule, which may be localised to the labia majora. It is unilateral and frequently vaguely linear. Lesions may extend into the inguinal fold and onto the leg.

In the perianal area, epidermal naevi of the vulva may have a warty or pedunculated appearance. This will give rise to friction symptoms from clothes and wiping. In some cases, the naevus may also be intractably itchy and unresponsive to topical anti-inflammatory agents.

Investigation

Vulval epidermal naevi, particularly when not obviously part of a larger linear lesion, are frequently mistaken for lichenified eczema or warts, and in children this may then lead to allegations of child sexual abuse. Biopsy will confirm the diagnosis and differentiate them from either eczema or HPV-related lesions.

Management

For symptomatic lesions, full-thickness localised excision is the best treatment. Partial treatment with such modalities as laser or shave excision is acceptable but may need to be repeated if the lesion recurs.

Many topical therapies have been advocated, including retinoids and calcipotriol, but our experience with them has been disappointing.

The most logical management is a combination of excision of symptomatic areas and reassurance for non-symptomatic ones.

Vulval Hyperpigmentation

Vulval hyperpigmentation is usually seen in dark-skinned patients and is normal. Similar to melanosis vulvae, it is asymptomatic but is of earlier onset. The difference from melanosis vulvae is that it is confluent rather than patchy, usually involving the outer surfaces of the labia minora.

Drugs that cause hyperpigmentation of the skin elsewhere may do the same on the vulva. The classic drug that does this is minocycline. A drug history should always be taken into account in any patient with acquired vulval hyperpigmentation.

Melanosis Vulvae

Melanosis vulvae is strictly speaking not an acquired lesion, but acquired hyperpigmentation of the vulva (Figure 7.7). This condition is very common but unusual before middle age.

The presentation is with multiple, discontinuous brown to black, well-defined macules on the labia minora and perineum. These lesions are not raised. They are invariably asymptomatic and noted at Pap test or accidentally by the patient.

Melanosis vulvae often cause concern because it comes into the differential diagnosis of vulval melanoma. However, melanoma is usually a single lesion as opposed to melanosis vulvae, which is usually multiple.

Histopathology of melanosis vulvae simply reveals increased melanin in the basal layer of the epidermis. There is no evidence of malignancy.

Management

If there is any doubt, particularly with a solitary lesion and to allay a patient's fears, a small biopsy makes this diagnosis. Once this is established, reassurance is all that is required.

Acanthosis Nigricans

Acanthosis nigricans (Figure 7.8) is an important condition to recognise as it has associations that have serious implications for the patient's health. These are mainly endocrine related and include obesity, insulin resistance, type 2 diabetes, polycystic ovarian disease and internal malignancy.

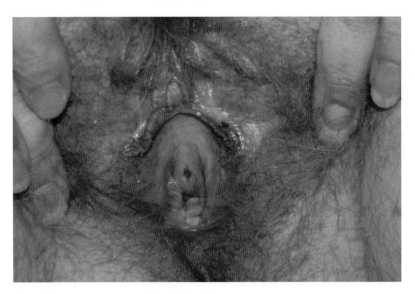

Figure 7.7 Benign vulval melanosis.

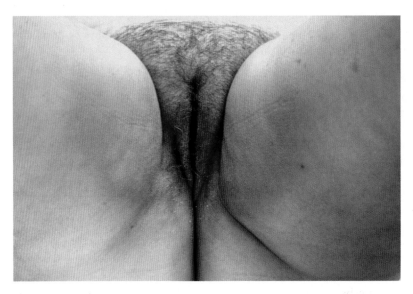

Figure 7.8 Acanthosis nigricans.

Presentation

Acanthosis nigricans is a skin condition that bilaterally affects the genital area and inner thighs, axillae and neck with a characteristic velvety hyperkeratotic thickening of the skin associated with hyperpigmentation. It may be associated with multiple skin tags and has a characteristic histopathology showing seborrhoeic keratosis-like thickening of the epidermis.

The difference between this condition and vulval hyperpigmentation is the presence of hyperkeratosis evidenced by thickening of the skin surface. It is rarely confined to the vulva and usually involves the inguinal folds and inner thighs, as well as other parts of the skin.

Management

A finding of acanthosis nigricans mandates a glucose-tolerance test and possible referral to an endocrinologist. In older patients where there is no obvious cause, a directed search for malignancy should be carried out.

Dowling–Degos Disease

This is a very rare condition but is included here because it comes into the differential diagnosis of acanthosis nigricans. Dowling–Degos disease is a genetic condition inherited in an autosomal-dominant fashion.

Presentation

It presents in adult life with multiple freckle-like lesions of the axillae and groins. The neck and other parts of the skin may also be involved. The pigmentation may also be reticulate or almost confluent.

It has a characteristic histopathology, which will differentiate it from acanthosis nigricans. It is important to do so because it is not associated with endocrinopathies or insulin resistance.

Management

There is no effective treatment, nor is any required.

Vulval Angiokeratomas

Vulval angiokeratomas (Figure 7.9) are vascular papules of the vulva. They are very common and are harmless.

Presentation

Patients present with multiple small red to purple papules on the labia majora. The onset of the lesions is from middle age and beyond. They are similar to Campbell de Morgan spots, which are usually found on the trunk. They become more common with advancing age. When they are dark purple, they may be confused with melanocytic lesions, and doctors and patients may be concerned about melanoma.

Very occasionally, these lesions may bleed if knocked or scratched, especially during a shower. Rarely, they may become much larger during pregnancy.

The histopathology is of a small haemangioma.

Patients may become anxious if the papules bleed and alarmed at what they might represent. Angiokeratomas are usually easy to diagnose clinically and, like seborrhoeic keratosis, there is a characteristic dermoscopic appearance.

Management

Reassurance is all that is required, but if any lesions are bleeding or causing discomfort, they can easily be ablated with simple diathermy or cryotherapy.

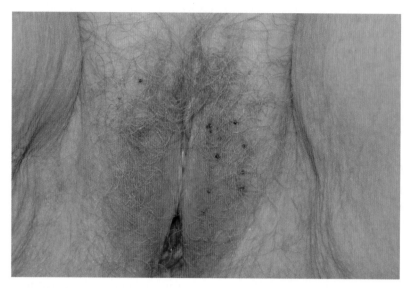

Figure 7.9 Angiokeratomas.

Vulval Lymphangiectases

These lesions are usually seen in patients who have had lymph node dissection and radiotherapy for a gynaecological malignancy and are the result of dermal fibrosis, which compresses the cutaneous lymphatics. They sometimes occur as the result of chronic bacterial cellulitis, or rarely Crohn's vulvitis.

Presentation

These lesions present as clear blebs, which may from time to time leak clear lymphatic fluid. There is often also associated firm oedema of the surrounding area.

Patients with lymphatic stasis are at risk of secondary infection, particularly with group A *Streptococcus*.

Management

Although there is nothing that needs to be done or indeed can be done for such lesions, patients should be warned to present immediately if they experience pain, redness, swelling or fever. These symptoms may represent cellulitis. Patients who have lymphangiectases as the result of chronic cellulitis will require long-term antibiotics.

Cysts, Boils and Things That Simulate Them

Sebaceous Cysts

These benign lesions are quite common on the vulva and are often multiple, involving the labia majora bilaterally (Figure 7.10). They appear at any age from adolescence on but are unusual in children. They become slowly more numerous with time. The lesions tend to occur at points of friction, especially in obese women.

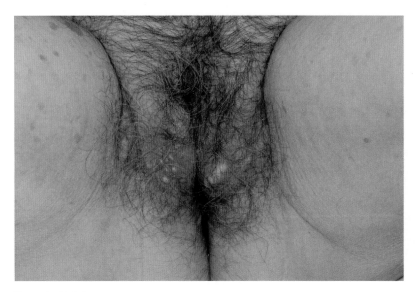

Figure 7.10 Sebaceous cysts.

Sebaceous cysts of the vulva are usually merely a cosmetic problem, but occasionally they may become inflamed and even secondarily infected. In these situations, they may rupture, extruding their contents. Patients often make their situation worse by deliberately squeezing these lesions.

Presentation

Sebaceous cysts appear as dermal nodules with a yellowish colour. They are ovoid, mobile and well defined. The size varies from a few millimetres to 20 mm. These cysts have a characteristic histopathology showing a unilocular lesion with a dermally located keratin-filled cyst. The cyst wall is an inpouching of the epidermis and therefore such cysts have a punctum, from which the malodorous contents of the cyst can usually be extruded.

Management

If a cyst is inflamed and painful, simply incising and draining it will relieve this. Antibiotics are sometimes necessary for infected lesions. Patients should modify their clothing if the distribution of cysts indicates a frictional aetiology, and must be warned never to squeeze these lesions.

There is, however, only one definitive treatment for sebaceous cysts and that is excision. On the vulva, these lesions are somewhat easier to remove than on the rest of the skin as the connective tissue is relatively loose. The cyst can usually be extracted through a small incision made over the lesion. Excision should be delayed for at least 3 months after a secondary infection, to minimise post-operative infection.

Our usual advice in uncomplicated cases is not to treat, but some patients are sufficiently concerned to seek surgery. The patient must understand that more cysts may form, and should be counselled about reducing heat, sweat and friction in this area.

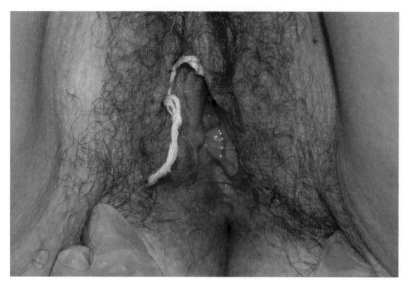

Figure 7.11 Boil.

Folliculitis and Boils

Folliculitis is a superficial *Staphylococcus aureus* infection of hair follicles. Boils are simply a deeper and more extensive form of folliculitis (Figure 7.11).

The vulva is prone to hair follicle infection because:

- It is a hair-bearing area
- It is a common site for chronic staphylococcal carriage
- Pubic and groin hair removal by waxing and shaving produces micro-abrasions on the skin that are easily infected
- Vulval skin may become macerated and overheated, which further increases the chances of hair follicle disruption due to heavy sweating

Presentation

Folliculitis presents with multiple superficial itchy pustules. Boils are larger and deeper, and both tender and painful. The two conditions may go together. Both tend to be very chronic because the underlying pathology is usually a staphylococcal carrier state, which has to be addressed in order to obtain a cure.

Investigation

Folliculitis can easily be confirmed with a simple bacterial swab. It is important to do this to prove the diagnosis and determine the sensitivity of the organism, and to exclude meticillin-resistant *S. aureus* (MRSA) carriage.

Management

Treatment involves the following:

- Drain any boils
- Treat the acute episode with appropriate oral antibiotics

- Use an antiseptic wash in the shower daily
- Hot wash all garments, sheets and towels for a month
- Stop waxing and shaving until the episode is over
- Ask about any symptoms in the patient's partner who may also require the same strategy; even if the partner is asymptomatic, they should also wash with an antiseptic at the same time
- If the patient resumes hair removal, recommend clipping rather than shaving or waxing
- If the patient wants to be permanently free of pubic hair, recommend laser hair removal

Inflammatory Tinea of the Pubic Area

Although very unusual, tinea (a dermatophyte infection) may cause a dramatic eruption of sudden onset involving the vulva and pubic area.

Presentation

It appears indistinguishable from a severe attack of boils and may present with swelling, inflammatory nodules and draining sinuses.

The clue that you are not dealing with a staphylococcal infection is a lack of response to antibiotics and negative swabs. The patient may own guinea pigs or other pets from which the infection is acquired.

Investigation

The diagnosis is made with a skin biopsy and culture of skin scrapings.

Management

Treatment is with an oral antifungal drug such as griseofulvin, itraconazole, fluconazole or terbinafine in the same doses and duration used to treat tinea of the scalp or beard.

Hidradenitis Suppurativa

This is a relatively common, chronic and recurrent condition of the vulva and other skin sites, the severity of which ranges from a mild nuisance to a disabling, life-ruining condition (Figure 7.12).

Hidradenitis suppurativa is a genetic disease that may run in families. It is rare in childhood and usually appears for the first time at or after puberty. This is because it is an androgen-sensitive condition that requires adult levels of this hormone to express itself.

For the same reason, it rarely appears after menopause. Despite the association with androgen, women with hidradenitis suppurativa have normal serum androgen levels. Their problem is at the end organ: the hair follicle, which is more sensitive than normal to androgenic stimulation.

It has been observed that cigarette smoking is a trigger in hidradenitis suppurativa, and it has been postulated that nicotine may be causative in some patients. It is also more common in obese patients.

Aetiology

The aetiology is thought to be a chronic inflammation of apocrine sweat glands, and it therefore is located on areas where these glands are present: the vulva, perianal area, buttocks,

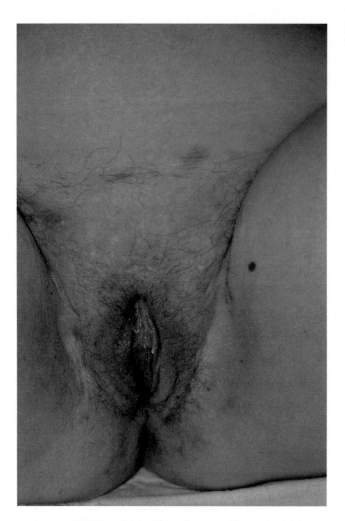

Figure 7.12 Hidradenitis suppurativa.

axillae and under the breasts. The exact pathogenesis is unknown. The currently accepted theory is that apocrine glands are easily blocked in these patients, which then rupture causing inflammation of surrounding tissue.

The disease is not an infection, and swabs may grow a variety of non-pathogenic bacteria, the treatment of which is ineffective.

Presentation

Hidradenitis suppurativa presents with tender painful nodules that drain pus, sinuses, pustules, abscesses and comedones. Lesions may be followed by significant scarring.

Patients often go without a diagnosis for many years, being thought to have a recurrent staphylococcal infection, even though swabs are consistently negative.

When hidradenitis suppurativa involves the vulva, the distribution is usually on the mons pubis, labia majora, inguinal folds, perianal area and buttocks.

Although it is more common in women than men, it is less severe. It may exacerbate pre-menstrually.

It may be associated with severe acne, pilonidal sinuses and a condition known as dissecting cellulitis of the scalp.

A number of severity assessment tools have been proposed. The earliest, devised in 1989, was the Hurley staging system, but there have been many since, most useful for clinical trials and studies. Severity does not always correlate well with the response to treatment.

Investigation and Diagnosis

As long as staphylococcal and fungal infection have been ruled out, the diagnosis is a clinical one. The finding of vulval comedones is pathognomonic: they occur in no other disease.

Hidradenitis suppurativa does not have a diagnostic histopathological appearance. A biopsy is generally not necessary to diagnose this condition, nor is it diagnostic.

The main differential diagnosis is recurrent staphylococcal boils. This can readily be ruled out by a bacterial swab from a new lesion. In hidradenitis suppurativa, swabs will not demonstrate *S. aureus*, or if they do, appropriate antibiotics will be ineffective.

Rare diseases that may come into the differential diagnosis, particularly with perianal disease, include atypical pyoderma gangrenosum, Crohn's disease and infections such as mycobacterial folliculitis. However, none of these will be characterised by comedones.

Management

Many patients arrive with a long history of recurrent episodes of minor surgery to drain or excise lesions and multiple short courses of antibiotics.

Our experience has been that, in most cases, treatment of this condition is straightforward. However, some patients are very challenging to treat.

Unfortunately, evidence for treatment is largely anecdotal because there is little high-quality research.

Medical Therapy

In mild cases, topical clindamycin 2% or erythromycin 2% with regular antiseptic washes may reduce symptoms, but systemic therapy tends to be much more effective.

If the patient smokes, she should make every attempt to stop. Obesity will exacerbate the suffering in this condition, but weight loss alone will not have a significant effect on the course of the disease.

Our usual first line of therapy is an oral anti-androgen.

If the patient is on the combined oral contraceptive pill, we change this to one with an anti-androgenic progestogen such as cyproterone acetate or drospirenone.

If the combined oral contraceptive pill is not indicated, the most cost-effective and safe treatment in our hands is spironolactone 100 mg/day. In resistant cases, the dose may be doubled. It is protocol to check serum potassium levels regularly, but it has recently been shown that this is not necessary in young, healthy women. Studies have shown anti-androgens to be more effective than antibiotic treatment, and we have observed that our own patients have similar results with anti-androgens alone compared with a combination of anti-androgens and antibiotics such as minomycin.

In the anti-androgen group of drugs, spironolactone has the advantage of being well tolerated and inexpensive. We find that it has high patient acceptance, and most are happy to continue on it long term given the disruption to quality of life that hidradenitis suppurativa can cause. In women where there is a risk of pregnancy, contraception must be advised as this drug may feminise a male fetus. It may also result in menstrual irregularity in those not on the oral contraceptive pill and has been associated with breast lumps and tenderness. Some women, particularly those with a low body mass index, may experience a drop in blood pressure at 100 mg/day and it is safest in these patients to commence at 50 mg/day and slowly increase the dose. In practice, we find that these adverse events are uncommon.

Other anti-androgens are:

- Cyproterone acetate 5–25 mg/day
- Finasteride 5 mg/day
- Dutasteride 0.5 mg/week
- Flutamide 250 mg/day

Other Treatments

- Intra-lesional steroid injections using triamcinolone 10 mg/ml into early lesions may abort individual attacks.
- Many authors advocate oral antibiotics; however, we find these relatively disappointing; a recent study showed that when used with or without spironolactone there was no difference in outcome.
- Oral and topical retinoids have been advocated in the medical literature, but we have found them disappointing.
- There are anecdotal reports of the use of immunosuppressants such as cyclosporin and methotrexate.
- There has been a case series of women treated with metformin.
- Recently tumour necrosis factor-α inhibitors such as infliximab and adalimumab have shown promise in treating patients with hidradenitis suppurativa that is either not controlled by anti-androgens, or where they are not tolerated or contraindicated. This is currently off label. These 'biological agents' are currently very expensive, but our experience with them so far has been positive. Referral to a dermatologist is recommended.

Unfortunately, this condition cannot be assumed to always remit at menopause and treatment may need to be life-long. Many patients are willing to accept this because of the severe morbidity imposed by untreated hidradenitis suppurativa.

Surgery

Acute painful lesions may be incised and drained, but marsupialisation has a much better effect. This should be followed by topical application of clindamycin 2% or erythromycin 2%. This is palliation, however, and not a cure.

Excisional surgery is curative and therefore the treatment of choice. However, this applies only to patients who have involvement in areas that can be widely excised without producing disfigurement. For patients with involvement of the labia, perianal skin or buttocks, this may not be a practical option.

There are many reports in the literature regarding extensive surgery and more recently CO_2 laser ablation to cure hidradenitis suppurativa.

These options come with the risk of major post-operative implications for wound healing, scarring and sexual function, and should be reserved for very severe cases.

Sebaceous Adenitis

This recently described condition involves the inner surface of the labia minora. It presents with recurrent tender and painful nodules, often flaring pre-menstrually. The nodules may drain purulent material.

Biopsy reveals inflammation of the sebaceous glands found on the labia minora. Unlike hidradenitis suppurativa, this condition does not scar, nor is it associated with comedones. It is found only on the mucosal surface of the labia minora.

The onset of this condition is in adult life, the mean age being mid-30s. The sebaceous gland contains androgen receptors, which are thought to be involved.

The differential diagnosis of such lesions includes bacterial infection. An infected Bartholin's cyst is easy to rule out because it arises in a different area. The recurrent and multiple nature of these lesions, once bacteriology has ruled out infection, differentiates it from both of these conditions.

Like hidradenitis suppurativa, this condition can be suppressed with topical macrolides and oral anti-androgens, including the oral contraceptive pill with an anti-androgenic pro-gestin. We have also used spironolactone successfully in this condition.

Vulval Neoplasia

Because the vulva is part of the skin, it is not surprising that the cancers that occur on the vulva are common skin cancers that occur elsewhere. These include:

- Basal cell carcinoma
- Vulval intra-epithelial neoplasia (squamous cell carcinoma *in situ*)
- Extra-mammary Paget's disease (Paget's disease that occurs on the vulva)
- Melanoma

Such lesions should be biopsied without delay.

When Should You Suspect That Your Patient Has a Vulval Cancer?

Any new lesion that appears suspicious or presents with a change in characteristics over time should be biopsied without delay. If there is genuine concern about melanoma, the lesion should be excised completely if possible.

Vulval Intra-Epithelial Neoplasia

Vulval intra-epithelial neoplasia (VIN) is the most common form of vulval neoplasia. Histopathologically, it is an *in situ* form of squamous cell carcinoma indistinguishable from what is known on sun-exposed skin as Bowen's disease. However, on the vulva, the most common aetiological factors are not sun but oncogenic genotypes of HPV and lichen sclerosus.

There is still much controversy about the classification and prognosis for VIN. It used to be thought that VIN could be graded in the same way as cervical intra-epithelial neo-plasia (CIN). This grading does not actually reflect the biological behaviour of VIN and should be abandoned. Clinically significant VIN is full-thickness neoplasia with invasive potential.

Gynaecological oncologists do not consider VIN to be a malignancy. Dermatologists might not agree with this, because they consider squamous cell carcinoma *in situ* of skin a malignancy no matter where the location, including the vulva. In fact, squamous cell carcinoma *in situ* of the vulva potentially carries more risk than its equivalent on sun-exposed skin, because if progression to invasive squamous cell carcinoma occurs, the risk for metastasis is greater on the vulva.

The current histopathological classification for VIN is unfortunately still very confusing (see Chapter 4) but divides VIN into two types:

- Usual VIN (uVIN), often associated with HPV and found in younger patients
- Differentiated VIN (dVIN), often associated with lichen sclerosus and found in older patients

Presentation

The presentation of VIN clinically is as papules and plaques, which may be any colour from white to brown. They may be solitary or multiple. Frequently, they have a warty, rough surface.

Other presentations include persistent raw or ulcerated areas. The lesions are frequently itchy, but this is not diagnostic or invariable.

It is more common in patients who smoke, who have genital and cervical warts, and are immunosuppressed, either by medication, inherited immunodeficiency or HIV disease. The HPV genotypes most often associated with VIN are the oncogenic types 16 and 18, also found in CIN and squamous cell carcinoma of the cervix.

The difference between VIN and invasive vulval squamous cell carcinoma relates histologically to whether the lesion has invaded below the basement membrane of the epidermis. Once this has happened, the prognosis of the lesion becomes much more guarded, and patients may require lymph node dissection in addition to wide local resection. Unlike squamous cell carcinoma of the skin, which rarely metastasises, squamous cell carcinoma of the vulva may do so. If vulval cancer spreads beyond the groin lymph nodes, the prognosis is grave.

Management

Details of treating this condition are beyond the scope of this book. The first step is to make a diagnosis by taking a biopsy of the lesion.

Further treatment includes surgery or laser treatment. In some cases, topical therapy with agents such as imiquimod may be used. Frequently, combinations of these agents are used, but despite this, recurrence occurs frequently.

Referral to a gynaecological oncologist is highly recommended.

Extra-Mammary Paget's Disease

This very uncommon condition is often confused with persistent dermatitis or psoriasis, and this is not surprising as this is what it superficially resembles (Figure 7.13). It is frequently a disease of older patients in their 70s and beyond.

The clue to diagnosis is that, although it appears to be a dermatitis, it is highly treatment resistant, with limited or no response to topical corticosteroids.

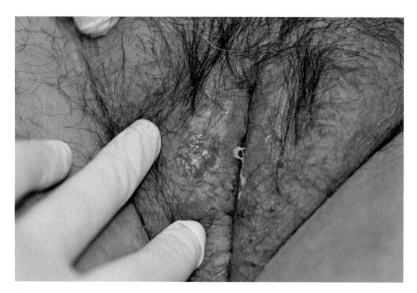

Figure 7.13 Extra-mammary Paget's disease.

Presentation

Patients usually complain of itch, soreness and swelling, or may present with the characteristic appearance but no symptoms.

There is often a plaque, which is usually red but may be pale, is either unilateral or bilateral, and may involve the vulva and/or perianal area. The edge of the plaque is usually better defined than an area of dermatitis and therefore may simulate psoriasis. The surface of the plaque may demonstrate a white scale that may look like 'icing sugar'.

Investigation

Extra-mammary Paget's disease has a very characteristic histopathology and a simple skin biopsy will make the diagnosis.

The condition may be associated with underlying malignancy of the bowel and bladder, and requires investigation. Immunohistochemical staining of the biopsy specimen may help to confirm the diagnosis and differentiate this risk.

Management

Treatment involves a combination of surgery and radiotherapy. Palliation with imiquimod may also be used, and recent studies support this in preference to surgery in cases where there is no invasive disease or underlying malignancy. Imiquimod therapy has to be prolonged, and many patients find it difficult to tolerate.

We recommend referral to a gynaecological oncologist.

Melanoma of the Vulva

Melanoma of the vulva is extremely rare. The appearance is no different from elsewhere on the skin, presenting with a slowly expanding red to brown to black lesion that may itch and bleed.

The hallmarks of melanoma include variation in colour, irregular shape and constant evolution. Lesions are often not symptomatic until they ulcerate.

Any suspected vulval melanoma should be excised with urgency and the patient referred to a tertiary referral centre for further management.

Acknowledgement

We would like to thank Dr Ken Jaaback MBBCh (Wits), FRANZCOG, CGO, Staff Specialist and Gynaecological Oncologist, John Hunter Hospital, Newcastle, NSW, Australia, for his help with this chapter.

Further Reading

Ali, H., Donovan, B., Wand, H., *et al.* (2013). Genital warts in young Australians five years into national human papillomavirus vaccination programme: national surveillance data. *British Medical Journal*, **346**, f2032.

Alikhan, A., Lynch, P. J. and Eisen, D. B. (2009). Hidradenitis suppurativa: a comprehensive review. *Journal of the American Academy of Dermatology*, **60**, 539–61.

Badr, D., Kurban, M. and Abbas, O. (2013). Metformin in dermatology: an overview. *Journal of the European Academy of Dermatology and Venereology*, **27**, 1329–35.

Chinniah, N. and Cains, G. D. (2014). Moderate to severe hidradenitis suppurativa treated with biologic therapies. *Australasian Journal of Dermatology*, **55**, 128–131.

Delport, E. S. (2013). Extramammary Paget's disease of the vulva: an annotated review of the current literature. *Australasian Journal of Dermatology*, **54**, 9–21.

Dixit, S., Olsson, A. and Fischer, G. (2014). A case series of 11 patients with hormone-responsive sebaceous adenitis of the labia minora. *Australasian Journal of Dermatology*, **55**, 80–3.

Garland, S. M., Insinga, R. P. and Sings, H. L. (2009). Human papilloma virus infections and vulvar disease development. *Cancer Epidemiology, Biomarkers and Prevention*, **18**, 1777–84.

Gormley, R. and Kovarik C. (2012). Human papillomavirus-related genital disease in the immunocompromised host. Part 1. *Journal of the American Academy of Dermatology*, **66**, 867–80.

Heller, D. (2007). Report of a new ISSVD classification of VIN. *Journal of Lower Genital Tract Disease*, **11**, 46–7.

Zouboulis, C., Desai, N., Emstestam, R., *et al.* (2015). European S1 guideline for the treatment of hidradenitis suppurativa/acne inversa. *Journal of the European Academy of Dermatology and Venereology*, **29**, 619–44.

Vulval Pain and Dyspareunia

Vulvodynia is a term that every doctor with an interest in vulval disease has heard of and read about. You will notice, however, that it is not the name of this chapter.

This is because vulvodynia is, by definition, a collection of symptoms, not a disease entity in itself.

Vulvodynia is in fact a poorly defined concept that simply means vulval pain. When your patient presents with vulval pain, you need to sort her into a meaningful diagnostic group. The management of each subtype is different. There is no single therapy that can be applied to all patients, yet the existing literature on the subject can give the impression that there is.

Vulvodynia is a term that was developed by the International Society for the Study of Vulvar Disease (ISSVD) in 1983. Their current definition is 'vulvar discomfort, most often described as burning pain, occurring in the absence of relevant visible findings or a specific, clinically identifiable neurologic disorder'.

The ISSVD has also produced a system of classifying vulval pain, where patients are categorised into those with an identifiable cause (A) and those that fit their case definition for vulvodynia (B). Within the latter group, pain is categorised as 'generalised' or 'localised' and classified as:

- Provoked: the pain is in response to friction, pressure, intercourse, insertion, etc.
- Unprovoked: the pain occurs spontaneously
- Mixed (provoked and unprovoked)
- Onset (primary or secondary)
- Temporal pattern

Despite the ISSVD's definition, doctors have diverse interpretations of the term vulvodynia and the literature on the subject can be confusing. Some clearly see it as vulval pain, some as itch, while others see it as vulval discomfort of any sort, and some see it as a disease in itself:

often one that they have had difficulty managing. In other words, the label is often applied inappropriately to any treatment-resistant vulval condition.

We prefer to avoid the term vulvodynia altogether. We refer to vulval pain, because it is simple, straightforward and does not carry with it the baggage of many years of medical confusion. If there is an observable lesion that is the cause for the pain, we call this 'lesional pain'. If there is no lesion, we call it 'non-lesional'.

We are, of course, at odds with many other authorities on the subject. We realise that there are websites and societies devoted to vulvodynia. However, our belief is that continuing to use this term, even though it is widely entrenched, will only prolong confusion on how best to manage the patient with vulval pain.

Pathophysiology of Vulval Pain

The mechanisms involved in vulval pain are still poorly understood. There are many reasons why the vulva is a pain-prone part of the body. These include:

- The complex anatomical structure of the bony pelvis and lower spine, and its vulnerability to damage
- The central position of the vulva and vagina within the pelvic myofascial complex, which facilitates pain referral from other pelvic viscera, specifically the uterus, bowel and bladder
- The fact that this area is subject to a great deal of physical stress: urination, menstruation, sexual intercourse, childbirth, defecation, and friction from clothes and pads
- Personal hygiene habits, which may inadvertently exacerbate the original problem
- The high levels of anxiety and fear that are often attached to problems involving the genital area
- The crucial importance of the genital area to a woman's sexual well-being and self-esteem

Nerve Supply to the Pelvis and Genital Area

Innervation to the vulva is provided by the pudendal nerve, which originates from S2–S4 nerve roots and the ilioinguinal and genitofemoral nerves, arising from L1–L2 (Figure 8.1). The two latter nerves are predominantly sensory, but the pudendal nerve contains motor, sensory and sympathetic fibres, which supply the complex autonomic reflexes of the pelvic organs. The epithelium of the vagina proper (i.e. deep to the hymenal ring) is not normally sensitive to pain.

The pudendal nerve supplies both the anal and urinary sphincters, whereas the muscles of the pelvic floor are mostly innervated via direct branches from the sacral plexus (S3–S5) with some input from the pudendal nerve, both voluntarily from higher centres in the brain and reflexly via the spinal cord.

It is known that there is a relationship between muscle function in the pelvis and pain, and studies have demonstrated that patients with pelvic pain have higher levels of resting muscle tone than other persons.

The convergence in the spinal cord of afferent impulses from viscera, skin and muscle can also lead to the phenomenon of referred pain. We are familiar with this when it comes to sciatica, but it is less well known that pain may also be referred to the vulva and distal vagina.

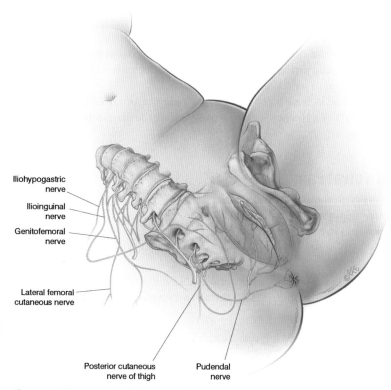

Iliohypogastric
nerve

Ilioinguinal
nerve

Genitofemoral
nerve

Lateral femoral
cutaneous nerve

Posterior cutaneous
nerve of thigh

Pudendal
nerve

Figure 8.1 Nerve supply of the vulva. With permission from Dr Levent Efe, CMI.

This convergence can also lead to alterations of sensation to nearby viscera, particularly the bladder. It is not uncommon for patients with vulval pain to complain of urinary frequency and urgency, lower abdominal pain and burning on urination.

Autonomic dysfunction may lead to loss of control of the vascular system of the vulva. The result is a variable degree of erythema of the vulval skin and the epithelium of the introitus. This is often misinterpreted as a rash and treated with cortisone creams. The vasoconstricting action of these medications is followed by a reflex vasodilatation, which may increase erythema and produce discomfort.

Chronic Pain

Pain sensation is mediated by three types of afferent nerve fibres: the large myelinated type Aβ fibres, which are responsible for touch, the smaller myelinated type A fibres, and the poorly myelinated or non-myelinated type C fibres. These latter fibres are responsible for pain perception, and the pain mediated by type C fibres in particular often has a burning quality. Type A fibres can, however, become involved in pain sensation, and when this occurs patients may develop allodynia. In this condition, stimuli that would normally elicit sensations of touch or pressure are perceived as pain. This explains why patients with vulval pain often find pressure from clothes difficult to cope with.

When patients experience chronic pain, afferent sensory processes mediated by type C peripheral nerve fibres via the dorsal horn spinal cord neurones appear to become sensitised, discharging more easily to lower levels of stimulation and at lower thresholds. They may even discharge spontaneously. This phenomenon has been termed 'wind-up'. There may be associated pathological changes in the dorsal horn connection and perhaps also in higher centres. It is helpful to understand this when there is no apparent noxious stimulus present. We also know that depressed and anxious patients have more problems with chronic pain, and that mental state is integral to pain experience.

It is important as a doctor to have a concept of how pain can occur in the absence of observable abnormality, particularly when it comes to explaining the diagnosis to the patient and indeed accepting it oneself.

Presentation of Vulval Pain

Broadly speaking, patients presenting with vulval pain tend to present either with something observable that explains their pain or with a normal-looking vulva.

They can be divided into two main groups:

- Pain that is directly attributable to an observable vulval or vaginal lesion or disease via cutaneous nociceptors: this is termed *lesional pain*
- Pain that is experienced in the absence of any observable vulvovaginal pathology and where the physical examination is normal for the patient's age and ethnic group: this is termed *non-lesional pain*

It must be remembered that the presenting symptoms may sometimes be due to *co-existing* lesional and non-lesional aetiologies.

Non-lesional Pain

We believe that the most likely explanation for non-lesional pain is neuropathy and/or referred pelvic muscular dysfunction. The source of this neuromuscular pain can include visceral pelvic problems such as prolapse, irritable bowel (particularly with chronic constipation), irritable bladder, uterine pain whether due to endometriosis or other pathology, or neuromuscular problems such as spinal or hip disease or dysfunction. A patient may have pain caused by both. Sometimes, a patient presents with pain that seems to have started with an episode of vulval skin disease (especially genital herpes or chronic thrush) but that persists after the skin problem has been resolved. Even though there has been a physical historical trigger for the pain, it should still be treated in this group.

Conversely, if a skin disease is present, it should always be considered initially as the cause of the patient's symptoms, even if this eventually proves not to be the case.

Non-lesional pain usually has the qualities of neuropathic pain. It is poorly localised and usually has a burning quality. It is spontaneous but can also be worsened by the sort of physical stimuli that would not normally cause pain, such as pressure from tight clothes or the application of topical therapy. There is a subgroup of non-lesional pain that is well localised. This tends to be more musculoskeletal in origin, rather than purely neuropathic.

Any form of chronic painful vulvovaginal or pelvic condition can predispose a patient to non-lesional pelvic pain. This includes period pain, bowel pain, chronic irritable bladder and any painful vulvovaginal condition. The reason is that chronic pain of any sort not only causes painful muscle spasm but also changes the way the brain perceives pain so that the threshold for experiencing pain becomes lower with time. This is called neuroplasticity.

Very occasionally, patients with psychiatric conditions can experience vulval pain as a symptom of their condition, and malingering patients may also sometimes complain of vulval pain. Our experience is that vulval pain due *primarily* to psychiatric disease is no more common than in any other part of the body.

Non-lesional pain has the following characteristics:

- It typically is best on first arising, becomes worse throughout the day, and is improved with rest at night.
- It is often positional: worsened by prolonged sitting and tight trousers.
- Hyperalgesia is characteristic of neuropathic pain and describes severe pain experienced from mild pain stimuli such as light touch. This can cause extra confusion because application of diverse topical therapies all seems to cause pain. This is inevitably attributed to the products themselves but is actually hypersensitivity to touch.
- Poor localisation of pain is often a feature of neuropathic pain. When asked to localise this sort of pain, patients are often unable to do so, and are only able to indicate the general area where the pain is experienced.
- Well-localised and especially unilateral pain is usually referred from the spine. Patients will localise a portion of skin on the affected side, but examination will show normal skin and no tenderness at this site.

When patients describe non-lesional vulvovaginal pain, they use the following words:

- Burning
- Rawness
- Dryness (even when on examination there is no evidence of it)
- Crawling
- Irritation
- Vulval awareness
- Itch or 'almost itch'
- Stabbing
- Pulsing
- Stinging

Lesional Pain

Pain due to an observable lesion or dermatosis is often caused by dermatological conditions that cause inflammation, ulceration, blisters, fissures and adhesions, and by conditions that cause vaginitis:

- It is frequently provoked by physical stimuli such as friction during intercourse or when inserting or pulling out a tampon, rubbing, scratching or wearing tight clothes.
- It is often accompanied by the symptoms of the causative dermatosis.
- It is usually bilateral.
- It is often worse during the night, when there are fewer external stimuli.
- It resolves promptly when the underlying condition resolves.

Lesional pain is usually well localised and has the familiar qualities of pain induced by injury.

Application of cream, which contain irritating substances such as preservatives, may sting. Changing from a cream to an ointment (which has no preservatives) usually solves this problem, and also helps to confirm that the pain is lesional.

This sort of pain resolves promptly when the underlying condition resolves.

When patients describe lesional pain they usually use the following words:

- Cut
- Split
- Tearing
- Sandpaper
- Sore

Which Skin Diseases of the Vulva Are Likely To Be Painful?

Dermatological conditions that affect the vulva tend to present with itch. Pain may be present, but it is usually sharp, easily localised pain that is due to excoriation from scratching or fissuring, which may occur in any dermatosis. Dyspareunia, if present, is usually due to friction involving raw areas.

Dermatological conditions that are predominantly painful rather than itchy are uncommon and include lichen planus, desquamative inflammatory vulvovaginitis, aphthous ulcers, erythema multiforme and fixed drug eruption. Bullous diseases such as bullous pemphigoid and cicatricial pemphigoid (see Chapter 5) can cause painful erosions but are extremely rare. Crohn's disease can present with painful erosions associated with oedema (see Chapter 5).

Vulval varicose veins may cause a dull ache, particularly after long periods of standing.

Infections such as genital herpes (see Chapter 5), vulval staphylococcal cellulitis and hidradenitis suppurativa (Chapter 7) are characteristically painful.

Atrophic vulvovaginitis tends to present with dyspareunia and a sensation of dryness (see 'Dyspareunia due to oestrogen deficiency' below).

Vaginal Dyspareunia

It is important to differentiate vaginal (superficial/entry) dyspareunia (felt in the vagina) from abdominal (deep) dyspareunia (felt in the abdomen). The first is usually caused by problems in the lower pelvis, and the second by problems in the upper pelvis or abdomen. There is widespread confusion about what constitutes 'deep' dyspareunia, with many doctors assuming this means 'deep in the vagina'. Our experience is that the important distinction is between *abdominal* as opposed to *vaginal* dyspareunia, and that it does not matter (in a diagnostic sense) how deep in the vagina it is felt. In the context of this book, we are discussing vaginal dyspareunia.

We find it most helpful to consider vaginal dyspareunia as a subset of vulval pain. Dyspareunia is usually primarily physical in origin, and therefore needs to be assessed in the context of the wider pelvis. Most often, it is part of a syndrome of non-sexual vulval pain, and it is the history of this background pain that will help in making a diagnosis. Dyspareunia can, however, occur as the only presenting symptom. In other words, the patient has no symptoms except pain during intercourse and/or tampon insertion.

Like more generalised vulval pain, vaginal dyspareunia may also be lesional or non-lesional. Lesional dyspareunia clearly occurs because the vulva and vagina is raw and inflamed.

Non-lesional dyspareunia occurs in the absence of any observable disease that could explain it. We believe that it is most often due to neuromuscular dysfunction. Rarely, it may be a somatoform disorder. This type of dyspareunia may be triggered by an underlying lesional disease but may remain long after the disease resolves. It may also appear in the absence of any lesional disease.

When discussing dyspareunia, it is important to explain pubococcygeal muscular dysfunction. This is found in many patients who have experienced vulval conditions that have caused dyspareunia for any reason. It can also occur as a primary problem in response to emotional stress and anxiety.

In this situation, the pubococcygeus muscle (the muscle that attaches anteriorly to the pubic bone and meets within the substance of the perineal body) goes into spasm as soon as any pressure is applied to the introitus. The patient describes a sharp, tearing sensation on intromission and immediate relief as soon as intercourse ceases. Tampon insertion often causes the same symptoms. It is unusual for this pain to linger for long after intercourse ceases unless there is also a lesion that has been irritated during intercourse.

Pubococcygeus muscle spasm is detectable on vaginal examination. It may be virtually impossible to insert an examining finger into the vagina because of this spasm, and any attempt to do so is described as severe pain by the patient. However, a patient who is relaxed with you as a doctor but apprehensive about intercourse may appear deceptively normal.

Lesional Group (nociceptive pain)

When dyspareunia is due to an ulcer or fissure, patients usually complain of the sort of pain that we would all experience if we cut a finger. This is known as 'nociceptive pain', in other words mediated by nociceptors in skin. This pain is usually well localised and is often accompanied by a small amount of bright post-coital bleeding. If the patient has a skin condition that is prone to fissuring, for example lichen sclerosus, this may occur as a result of intercourse. In this situation, the pain may not be immediate but may develop during intercourse. It then typically lasts for several days, until the fissure has healed.

Dyspareunia due to local physical causes usually improves promptly when the underlying dermatological condition is healed. However, it must be recognised that by the time effective treatment for the dermatosis is initiated, it may have caused secondary pubococcygeus muscle dysfunction that continues to cause dyspareunia.

Non-lesional Group (non-nociceptive pain)

In these patients, there is often a background of poorly localised or unilateral vulval pain. Some patients with non-lesional vulval pain deny dyspareunia but say they no longer want to have sex due to low libido or fear of being hurt. Those who do experience dyspareunia are usually either experiencing hyperalgesia or the same secondary pubococcygeus muscle dysfunction that occurs in patients with nociceptive pain.

Dyspareunia due to Oestrogen Deficiency (atrophic vaginitis)

Atrophic vaginitis is due to oestrogen deficiency and may present with dyspareunia alone, which patients often correctly identify as being associated with dryness. These women are lactating, post-menopausal or very thin.

Some patients, particularly those with a tendency to dermatitis elsewhere or who are atopic, may also develop a mild dermatitis of the introitus and labia minora. They may then complain of itching or irritation.

Post-menopausal women, who are prone to the vulvovaginal effects of post-menopausal oestrogen deficiency, are however also the group who may suffer from neuropathic vulval pain. As a result, an observation of atrophy may not be the cause of their vulval pain.

Examination

Examination shows a pale mucosa, with little lubrication and loss of normal rugosity. In younger lactating patients, however, there may be little to see other than a somewhat dry surface.

Management

Management should be initiated with topical treatment using oestrogen cream or pessaries, initially daily for 2 weeks and then twice weekly. Long-term use will be required if a beneficial response is achieved.

If dermatitis is present, hydrocortisone 1% ointment twice daily should be used concurrently, and the patient should use a soap substitute. Bland emollients and non-irritating lubricants during intercourse are helpful adjuncts to treatment. This condition should respond promptly to topical oestrogen cream or pessaries within a month. If there is no response, consider an alternative cause for the dyspareunia.

Approach to the Patient with Constant Vulval Pain

History Taking

Most patients with vulval pain will not volunteer the symptoms that help to make a diagnosis. They will, for example, complain about 'reduced libido' instead of dyspareunia; similarly, a patient is unlikely to volunteer that her vulval pain started during an episode of acute generalised psoriasis. A careful and comprehensive history is therefore essential, and should include the following:

- Duration of current episode of pain
- History of similar pain previously
- Historical triggers
    - Exacerbating/relieving factors
    - Associated symptoms, e.g. itch, vaginal discharge
    - History of skin disease, either vulval or elsewhere
    - History of menstrual pain
    - History of bladder pain
    - History of irritable bowel or chronic constipation
    - History of hip and/or back pain or injury
    - Leisure activities such as cycling, horse riding, skating
- Pain descriptors:
    - Sharp/dull/burn/sting/formication/stabbing
    - Associated itch, bleeding or abnormal vaginal discharge

- Continuous or episodic:
  - Length of episodes
  - Triggers for episodes
- Pain location:
  - On/within the labia majora
  - Central
  - Bilateral/unilateral
  - Anterior/posterior
  - Referral patterns
- Previous treatments:
  - Effective
  - Ineffective
- Impact on quality of life/sex/relationships

Systems Review

Because this type of pain is often referred, a complete systems review should be undertaken. Of particular importance is disease, dysfunction or injury to the lumbosacral spine, lower intestinal tract and anus, and lower limbs. This is because pain referral in the lower pelvis is usually *posterior to anterior*.

The systems review should include:
- Bladder: irritable bladder, recurrent infection, dysfunctional voiding
- Menstrual cycle/period problems
- Bowel problems: irritable bowel, constipation
- Musculoskeletal review:
  - Congenital problems
  - Injury
  - Orthopaedic/neurosurgical operations
  - Sciatica/other neuralgic leg symptoms
  - Orthotics ever worn
  - Foot/knee problems

Examination

Remember the golden rule: first exclude dermatological or infective causes.

Most of the patients referred to us because of vulval pain have a dermatological or infective cause that has been previously overlooked. We even see patients referred from sex therapists, who have realised that the woman in front of them does not have a psychological or relational problem. The prevalence of these missed diagnoses means that most articles on 'vulvodynia' mistakenly include many women who do not have true non-lesional vulval pain. This confusion is, again, why we prefer not to use this term.

Conversely, there are patients with observable skin disease in whom the skin disease is not responsible for their symptoms. Nonetheless, a trial of treatment for the observed skin condition must be undertaken to ensure that it has been confidently excluded as the sole cause for the pain. In these patients, dermatological treatment will only be partially helpful.

Effective therapy is only possible after an accurate diagnosis has been made.

Having excluded dermatological or infective causes for vulval pain, the presentations can be divided into two groups:

1. Pain on insertion only.
2. Constant or intermittent pain not just related to insertion (although this may or may not be present as well).

Patients with vulval pain are rarely so uncomfortable that they are unable to be examined, but they may experience severe tenderness around the vestibule and in the vagina. It is often not possible to perform a speculum examination.

The most common local physical finding that causes acute vulval pain is a fissure. Fissuring may occur in almost any vulval dermatosis. The typical location is at 6 o'clock on the introitus. Even the tiniest fissures at the introitus may cause severe dyspareunia, so it is important to look closely, especially in vulval sulcae, and to gently stretch the skin. Usually, there is an accompanying vulval rash such as dermatitis, candidiasis, psoriasis or lichen sclerosus. However, occasionally patients develop persistent vulval fissuring in the absence of an obvious cause.

Surgical and obstetric scarring often make it difficult to distinguish between normal and abnormal appearances on genital skin. An assessment by an experienced gynaecologist may be necessary in these cases.

The most important questions to have in mind during the examination are:

- Is there a rash or lesion?

  o Look very closely for tiny fissures by gently stretching the skin.
  o If there is a visible abnormality, is it able to account for the patient's symptoms?
  o If there is some abnormality, is this simply a normal variant or consistent with the patient's age and ethnic group (for example, small labia minora in an elderly woman or pigmentation in a dark-skinned woman)?

- Where is the pain?

  o Is the pain unilateral or bilateral?
  o Does the pain radiate, for example to the groins?
  o Can the patient localise the pain?
  o Is there tenderness out of proportion to the degree of pressure exerted (we find it helpful to lightly touch the leg and at the same time touch the vestibule and ask the patient to compare the sensation)?
  o Is there any introital muscle spasm on digital vaginal examination? This is indicated by tightness, resistance and pain on gentle downward pressure at 6 o'clock in the posterior vaginal introitus.

- Does it relate to any observable abnormality or not?

If you have been reading other literature on dyspareunia, you may have noticed reference to the use of a cotton-tipped swab ('Q-tip'). We do not use this instrument, as we have found that it may actually cause pain. Furthermore, its use cannot distinguish between tenderness of the skin or of underlying structures. We find that the educated finger is more helpful.

Colposcopic examination after the application of acetic acid will make *any* inflammatory dermatosis appear white and is therefore diagnostically unhelpful, unless neoplasia is suspected. Its application usually provokes intense pain, and we believe that it is contraindicated in this setting.

Classifying Patients Who Have Non-lesional Vulval Pain

Neuropathic Pain

This is the most common aetiology in this category. The typical patient is a middle-aged to elderly woman who complains of a constant poorly localised burning sensation in the vulva. The pain is least severe in the morning after rest in bed and builds up during the day, especially with physical activity. Certain positions may be more uncomfortable than others, particularly sitting. The pain is not always associated with dyspareunia, but most patients develop a distaste for sexual intercourse because of it. This sensation is often not severe. It rarely wakes patients at night. However, it is constant and exhausting.

Some patients also complain of bladder symptoms such as urgency and frequency. When questioned, they often also have low back pain or sciatica, or have had a spinal disc protrusion.

When patients are examined, there is often no abnormality other than some degree of atrophy consistent with their age. However, atrophy alone does not cause burning pain. Erythema is often noted and may relate to loss of sympathetic control of skin vasculature. However, many patients have been treated with strong topical steroids for months in an attempt to treat the pain. This also causes erythema.

When you ask your patient to indicate the painful area, she will often indicate a horseshoe shape involving the perineum, introitus and lower labia majora bilaterally. It may radiate to the groin or inner thighs. In some patients, the discomfort is unilateral or even confined to one small spot, usually on the mucosal surface of the labia minora. In some patients, the area affected is periclitoral.

We believe that patients with this problem have neuropathic pain. The cause is still not understood.

Management

Medical Therapy

Like other forms of neuropathic pain, it is possible to obtain relief using oral medication. The most effective ones include:

- Tricyclic antidepressant medication: 10–50 mg amitriptyline or nortriptyline at night. We find amitriptyline more effective but nortriptyline is better tolerated.
- Doxepin 10–30 mg at night appears to be useful in patients whose main complaint is itch.
- Pregabalin 75 mg at night initially, increased to 75 mg twice daily. If tolerated, then increased gradually up to 300 mg twice daily, depending on the response.
- Gabapentin 100 mg at night initially, increased to 100 mg twice daily, and then slowly increased up to 600 mg three times daily. Again, the eventual dose depends on the clinical response.

It is very important when commencing tricyclic antidepressants to start with a very low dose of 5 mg at night and slowly increase it, so as to minimise side effects. It is important to explain that side effects usually pass and not to increase the dose beyond a level that they can tolerate. Although many texts advocate the use of high-dose tricyclics, in our experience if the drug does not work at low dose it is unlikely to work at high dose, and the side effects rapidly become intolerable.

The side effects of tricyclics include drowsiness, disorientation, dry mouth, blurred vision, constipation, hypotension and conduction defects causing palpitations. They should not be used in patients with narrow-angle glaucoma.

Many patients have great difficulty with the fact that these drugs are also used as anti-depressants. A statement we often hear is 'I don't want to be a pill popper'. It is important to explain that you are not using the drug as an antidepressant but as a pain reliever, and to mention that it is also used for migraine and bowel pain. Patients are often very apprehensive about taking such medication, and any side effect will cause them to give up quickly. They need to be encouraged to persevere as it is usually the initial 2 weeks that are the most difficult.

Gabapentin and pregabalin may be combined with low-dose tricyclics.

If a medication is effective, most patients who respond will notice obvious, if small, improvements in their pain within 4–6 weeks. The dose should then be increased slowly until no more pain is felt. This can take up to 1 year, although some patients feel better very quickly. Once the pain has been relieved, it may be necessary for the patient to remain on their medication indefinitely, although an attempt is usually made to reduce it once the pain has been adequately controlled for some months.

At the time of writing, we do not believe that there is sufficient evidence for the use of compounded topical neuromodulating agents. Amitriptyline applied topically is a local anaesthetic but has much more potential for side effects than xylocaine. An integral part of the effect of neuromodulating drugs is on spinal neurological function, which topical agents cannot change. Furthermore, topical agents may cause hypersensitivity reactions, and they are expensive.

Exercise

Rest is an important component of treating this condition. Once patients feel better, they often become much more active than before, and this can cause the pain to become worse again.

On the other hand, carefully supervised exercises that strengthen the lower back, as well as weight loss, can make a big difference and eventually allow withdrawal of medication. We recommend this if the patient is well enough and young enough, particularly with the help of a physiotherapist.

We see young women, however, who exercise so much that their core and pelvic floor become too toned and tight. These individuals often require down-training of their muscles to improve vulval pain.

Complementary Medicine, Counselling and Explanation

Some patients appear to benefit from acupuncture and chiropractic, and some find that counselling is helpful, particularly if the counsellor has expertise in chronic pain management.

In some patients, an explanation of what is happening is all they need. The pain is not severe and they would rather live with it than take medication.

Neuropathic vulval pain is much better recognised than it has been in the past, and neuropathic pain in general has started to receive much more attention in the medical literature. It is important not to dismiss a patient with chronic vulval pain just because they appear normal. If they apparently have a skin condition and topical treatment is not effective within a reasonable time, consider the possibility of neuropathic pain as the real cause of their problem.

Referred Pain

The nerve supply to the vulva originates from the L1–L2 and S2–S4 nerve roots (see Figure 8.1) via the pudendal and genitofemoral nerves. Compression or injury to these nerves may result in pain referred to the vulva, similar to sciatica.

Presentation

There is much overlap between this problem and neuropathic pain, but in this situation the pain is often well localised, unilateral or much more pronounced on one side; it may have a shooting, electric shock stabbing or cramping component, and may have been of sudden onset. The patient is often much younger, and may present from early in the third decade of life.

History Taking

When questioned, these patients may also give a history of low back pain or sciatica, and may have a history of a back injury from lifting, falling off a horse, a skiing or motor vehicle accident, or falling on the coccyx. Episodes of vulval pain can be associated with low back pain.

This sort of pain typically also has a burning quality in exactly the same way as neuropathic pain.

Management

It is important to rule out gross spinal pathology, although this is very unusual in our patients. Management of any anorectal problems is also essential.

Management of this type of pain is ideally with a physiotherapist who is skilled in both the pelvis and spine. Neuromodulating drugs may be necessary. General measures such as lifestyle modification and weight loss will help.

Role of Physiotherapy

Physiotherapy is an essential element of treating many patients with non-lesional vulval pain. In these patients, retraining of the pelvic floor muscles will reduce resting muscle tone and in turn reduce dorsal horn sensitivity. The role of physiotherapy is either as an alternative to medication or to allow an eventual withdrawal of medication. It has high levels of patient acceptance, and the psychological support of the physiotherapist should not be underestimated. We recommend this if the patient is well enough and young enough to embark on it.

The physiotherapy history is similar to the medical history. Physical examination, however, concentrates on the musculoskeletal components of the spine, pelvis and lower limbs. A gentle but thorough assessment may take more than one session, due to the high levels of anxiety and fear in this patient group.

Resting tone, trigger points and pain scores of pelvic floor, hip and relevant spinal muscles are assessed, as well as the presence or absence of prolapse and any apparent fascial defects.

A more generalised musculoskeletal assessment is also performed including assessment of gait and posture, generalised muscle tone and breathing patterns, and specific examination of the lumbar spine and pelvic girdle, plus identification of any trigger points in the abdominal, hip, gluteal and back muscles.

Education is an important first step in physiotherapy management. A clear explanation of the possible causes of their pain and the nature of chronic pain is essential. Behaviour and lifestyle modification such as correct posture, good back care, good bladder and bowel habits, vulval hygiene, avoidance of aggravating factors, stress reduction, and incorporation of appropriate general exercise and relaxation activities/techniques into daily life is important.

Physical techniques aim to increase awareness and proprioception, normalise tone, improve muscle discrimination and relaxation, desensitise and increase tissue elasticity, and reduce the fear of vaginal penetration. Techniques may include myofascial massage and trigger point release. Use of vaginal dilators may be employed both during sessions and as part of the patient's home programme. Once normalisation of resting pelvic floor muscle tone had been achieved, further attention may need to be directed to strength, endurance, coordination and timing of these muscles.

Treatment of co-existing lumbar spine and sacroiliac joint dysfunction via joint mobilisation and muscle energy techniques is often necessary.

Somatoform Disorder

Until recently, vulval symptoms were considered to be mainly psychological in origin. In our practice, this is an uncommon cause of chronic vulval pain.

Patients with psychogenic pain are a very difficult group to diagnose and, in many cases, impossible to treat. It takes experience to recognise this condition, and even so it is inevitably a diagnosis of exclusion.

Presentation

Typically, the complaint is of constant pain, often with a burning quality, that does not fit easily with physical pain patterns. There is a bizarreness to the descriptions, which may change with each consultation. The pain is often not confined to the vulva and may generalise to involve the whole body.

Patients with psychogenic pain rarely come to the consultation alone. They are brought in by relatives who are desperate for an end to the misery that the patient inflicts on other family members. Often, they have seen numerous doctors and are angry and frustrated. When they do come by themselves, they often remark that their family has insisted that they see you.

Examination

When one attempts to examine such patients, they may be quite uncooperative.

This type of patient experiences pain as a manifestation of an underlying psychiatric illness. They may have a conversion disorder or may be malingerers who derive secondary gain from their problem by manipulating those around them, particularly their relatives. Malingerers do not wish to recover, as the pain is a way of satisfying their needs. It is their relatives who want a cure.

We occasionally see patients with this sort of pain who are engaged in a court case to sue a person whom they feel is responsible for their pain. Some have appeared to recover after their legal action is resolved.

Management

These patients derive secondary gain from their pain and do not wish to recover. For this reason, this is a very difficult situation to treat. They need the help of a psychiatrist, but this is one doctor that these patients usually flatly refuse to see. They medicalise their problem, and as soon as they encounter a doctor who refuses to legitimise their medical model, they seek help elsewhere. It is their relatives who want a solution.

Our approach is to help the relatives cope with the patient. It is best for both if the secondary gain is truncated. Unfortunately, the relatives are often unwittingly part of the problem, and patience and persistence are needed to convince them of the real nature of the illness.

Sexual Abuse

Many studies have demonstrated that 20–25% of women can recall sexual abuse as a child or adolescent. It has been shown that sexual abuse is associated with a lifetime risk of psychiatric disease and somatoform symptoms, drug abuse, phobia, depression and panic disorder. Child sexual abuse has been correlated with chronic pelvic pain, but the question of whether this is a major factor in subsequent dyspareunia is unknown.

Childhood sexual abuse is a broad term that includes any exposure to sexual acts and does not always imply penetration, particularly in young children. It is seen in all counties and social classes, and the perpetrators are usually known to and trusted by the child.

You should of course include sexual abuse as a possible aetiology for vaginal dyspareunia. However, it is best mentioned further on in the history taking, when you have the sense that you have built up a trusting relationship with your patient. Many patients do not wish to talk about or admit to it, and they may have forgotten about it, so any questioning about it is inherently problematic. Furthermore, an answer in the affirmative cannot be assumed to explain the patient's problem.

With regard to non-lesional vulval pain where there appear to be clear non-sexual triggers, delving into childhood sexual abuse may simply alarm or upset your patient and not contribute to management. In our practice, we enquire about this only if there are no other obvious causes.

The Depressed or Obsessive Patient with Vulval Disease

Depressed patients may also experience pain as a manifestation of their depression. This may present as psychogenic pain alone, but a more common scenario is a patient with an uncomfortable vulval condition who copes poorly due to a concurrent depressive illness.

As a result, a physical condition that would normally be mildly painful is experienced as excruciating, and the most common term that such patients use to describe themselves is 'in agony'. This is characteristic of the catastrophising that often happens in depression.

Patients with obsessive–compulsive disorder may also find vulval conditions extremely difficult to cope with. Washing rituals may further irritate their skin. They may become irrationally focused on infection, particularly genital herpes, and they may experience great difficulty touching themselves to apply creams or insert tampons.

They may insist on wearing pads and liners at all times because they feel this is hygienic, which further exacerbates their skin problem. As a result, they may find themselves in a vicious cycle. Not surprisingly, anxiety and depression commonly worsen.

Presentation

Unlike patients with a somatoform disorder who are commonly angry, these patients present as sad and anxious. Even when they lack insight into their condition, they are usually receptive to the suggestion of psychiatric help and antidepressant medication.

Any patient with a long-standing vulval problem, particularly where pain is part of the symptomatology, may become depressed, and the depression will exacerbate the pain. For many patients, the concept of long-term control of a condition that cannot be cured is very hard to accept.

Dyspareunia and Pain on Tampon Insertion Without any other Abnormalities

In a patient with dyspareunia, it is first important to rule out a physical cause. However, if vaginal bacteriology is normal, there is no oestrogen deficiency and physical examination (including careful examination for fissures) is normal, we believe that this is due to muscle spasm in response to any attempt at insertion into the vagina.

Examination

It has been found that patients with this problem have a high resting muscle tone in the pelvic floor, as measured on surface electromyography. They experience severe pain in response to stimuli that would ordinarily be experienced as touch, pressure or stretch.

This can usually be appreciated on digital examination. In a relaxed patient, it is possible to insert a finger into the vagina without encountering resistance. In the typical patient with muscle spasm, your finger will meet with firm resistance and the patient will experience pain from even light pressure.

Management

In this setting, oral tricyclic antidepressants and other drugs used to treat neuropathic pain are in our experience relatively ineffective.

Many articles in the medical literature suggest that patients with entry dyspareunia require psychotherapy. This is not true in everyone, and such a referral should be made on a case-by-case basis.

In patients with an anxious personality, relationship problems or a history of sexual abuse, such referrals are an essential part of management. However, many just require concrete advice on how to overcome muscle spasm and quickly overcome their problem. In our experience, psychotherapy alone without the pelvic floor advice is doomed to failure.

It is not known whether the pain causes the muscle spasm or vice versa, but expert pelvic physiotherapy can relieve this pain and often makes it possible for these patients to overcome their problem.

There are many pelvic floor physiotherapists who understand this type of dyspareunia and treat it effectively. These are our first line of management and one that patients welcome.

It is important to explain the mechanism and reassure very strongly and positively that this condition can be overcome with straightforward physiotherapy. We explain the nature of spinal reflexes such as the knee-jerk response and find that patients can easily relate to this.

Patients who appear to have developed this as a result of a skin condition should be warned at the outset that their dyspareunia may not resolve as quickly as their other symptoms.

There are patients in whom the prognosis has to be very guarded indeed. This group has primary dyspareunia, have never been able to insert anything into the vagina without severe pain and are angry, resentful and frustrated; they have invariably seen numerous doctors without improvement. They have had the problem for many years, have failed physiotherapy entirely, and it seems that their condition serves a purpose in their lives, albeit a dysfunctional one.

Interestingly, they usually have partners who support them and come with them to one doctor's appointment after the other. In this difficult-to-manage group, the possibility of a somatoform disorder (see above) has to be considered. However, this is not easy to prove. It is possible that these patients may benefit most from a long, supportive, therapeutic relationship with a doctor.

Surgical Treatment for Vulval Pain

There are three surgical approaches that have been advocated in the medical literature:

- Fenton's procedure, where the superficial muscles of the posterior introitus are incised to increase its dimensions
- Vestibulectomy, where the sensitive area of the introitus is excised, and the lining of the vagina is undermined and advanced to cover the area
- Intra-muscular botulinum toxin

Fenton's procedure is a very old operation, which is based on the notion that introital muscle tightness can be overcome surgically. It can be useful for the excision of persistent fissuring of the introital skin, where all other treatments have failed. However, we do not see it as a solution for muscle spasm.

The rationale for vestibulectomy is that the inside of the vagina is not sensitive to pain, and replacing sensitive introital skin with vaginal lining will eradicate the trigger point that sets off the muscle spasm. Advocates of this procedure claim a very high success rate where all other treatments have failed. The difficulty is that patients in these studies may have been characterised as having 'vulvodynia' without being further categorised and are therefore a heterogeneous population. In our practice, we have never needed to resort to this procedure. We are of the opinion that vestibulectomy may not be necessary when an accurate diagnosis leads to effective (non-surgical) treatments.

Intra-muscular botulinum toxin, which is injected directly into the levator ani muscle, is used to temporarily paralyse the muscle that is in spasm and causing the pain. It does appear to be effective as an adjunct to physiotherapy, enabling patients who have a great deal of trouble releasing the pelvic floor to progress with exercises. This therapy is still in an experimental stage. The effect lasts about 3 months, and the injections have to be repeated. Side effects include the possibility of urinary and faecal incontinence, and the cost is not inconsiderable. At this stage, we still see it as something to be considered when more conservative therapy has failed.

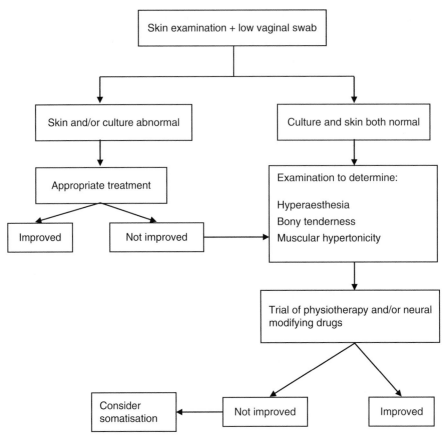

Figure 8.2 Diagnostic algorithm for vulval pain.

Diagnosing Vulval Pain

Diagnosis of vulval pain should follow the algorithm shown in Figure 8.2:

- Take a detailed history to determine:
  - The nature and timing of the pain
  - Whether the pain is associated only with intercourse or is present at other times
- Examine the patient to determine whether:
  - There is a lesion, fissure or rash
  - The vulva is essentially normal
- Investigations:
  - Take a low vaginal swab in every case
  - Biopsy may be required
- Treat any objective abnormality
- If the vulva appears normal and swabs are negative, the patient is likely to fall into one of the following groups:
  - Introital hyperalgesia: pain only with intercourse

- ○ Neuropathic pain: bilateral constant burning
- ○ Referred pain: burning pain, more pronounced on one side, history of back injury
- ○ Somatisation disorder: bizarre history and emotional state

Acknowledgement

We would like to thank Dr Newman L. Harris MBBS MMed (Pain Mgmt) FRANZCP FFP-MANZCA, Specialist in Pain Medicine and Consultant Psychiatrist, University of Sydney Pain Management and Research Centre, Royal North Shore Hospital, St Leonards, NSW, Australia, and Ms Tracey Cragg B.Sc. Grad. Dip. Phty. M.A.PA., Senior Women's Health Physiotherapist, Royal North Shore Hospital, St Leonards, NSW, Australia, for their help in preparing this chapter.

Further Reading

Damsted-Petersen, C., Boyer, S. C. and Pukall, C. F. (2009). Current perspectives in vulvodynia. *Women's Health*, **5**, 423–36.

Fischer, G. (2004). Management of vulvar pain. *Dermatologic Therapy*, **17**, 134–49.

Helme, R. (2014). Pharmacological management of neuropathic pain. *Pain Management Today*, **1**, 18–22.

Ponte, M., Klemperer, E., Sahay, A. and Chren, M. M. (2009). Effects of vulvodynia on quality of life. *Journal of the American Academy of Dermatology*, **60**, 70–6.

Vulval Disease in Children

When a pre-pubertal girl presents with an itchy or sore vulval rash, she is usually assumed to have thrush or a urinary tract infection. Poor hygiene or sexual abuse may also be considered. In fact, none of these is likely to be true.

Candidiasis does not occur in pre-pubertal girls, urinary tract infections do not result in rashes unless prolonged incontinence is present, sexually abused children rarely have physical signs, and overzealous hygiene is more likely to produce a rash than lack of hygiene.

Vulval disease in children is less common than in adults, and although many of the vulval diseases that affect adults also affect children, there are some important differences between the two groups. In both adults and children, dermatitis, psoriasis and lichen sclerosus are the most common dermatoses causing a chronic vulval rash. However, acute, recurrent and chronic candidiasis, which are important components of adult vulval disease, are not seen in the non-oestrogenised vulva and vagina of the child.

Birthmarks, particularly haemangiomas, of the vulva are an important issue in children, but in adults they have resolved long ago or have been diagnosed. Fusion of the labia is a self-limiting condition seen in small children, but in adults is seen only in the setting of lichen sclerosus or severe lichen planus.

Infective vaginitis is rare in children. Group A β-haemolytic streptococcal vulvovaginitis is a disease that occurs in children but in adults it is seen only sporadically.

Sexual abuse is always an issue to be considered in any genital presentation in children, but in fact is rarely a cause of vulval disease.

Older articles often blame paediatric vulval disease on the theory that non-oestrogenised pre-pubertal vulva skin must be fragile and sensitive. In fact, there is no evidence to support this. The incidence of vulval skin disease in children is much lower than in adults, and this implies that their vulval skin is less prone to disease. The use of oestrogen creams as a speculative treatment in this setting therefore has no basis in fact. Indeed, oestrogen creams are often very irritating when applied to children's skin.

The low-oestrogen environment of a child's vulva is physiological, not pathological. In fact, oestrogenisation in adult women is a liability that predisposes to vaginitis, particularly candidiasis.

Another common assertion is that vulval disease in children is due to poor hygiene and faecal contamination. This is a facile statement that is poorly evidenced and which trivialises and stigmatises this problem. In fact, mothers of small girls, particularly those with a vulval problem, are usually highly conscientious about genital hygiene and are more likely to be doing too much washing, rather than too little.

Parents often arrive in your office in a state of defensive high anxiety. They are embarrassed, ashamed, worried that they have an abnormal child and frustrated with treatment that has been ineffective. They may be harbouring fears of child abuse and mortified by their child having been sent home from school because of scratching behaviour.

What Causes Itchy Rashes in Pre-pubertal Children?

The common causes of rashes of the vulva comprise the usual dermatoses of the pre-pubertal age group: dermatitis and psoriasis, as well as the rare condition lichen sclerosus.

Dermatitis

Most who suffer from vulval dermatitis, both adults and children, are atopic.

The vulval skin of babies is remarkably resistant to disease, even though they are in nappies (diapers). Babies who suffer from atopic dermatitis rarely have signs of it in the well-hydrated skin under the nappy, and the onset of vulval dermatitis is often delayed until the child is out of nappies.

The resistance of genital skin appears to be lost in the older child, where the ongoing wearing of nappies, for example overnight in those with enuresis, starts to cause problems with irritant dermatitis similar to incontinent adults who wear absorbent garments.

Irritant contact dermatitis may occur as a result of contact with faeces, and this will most often happen in the context of the child with diarrhoea or chronic constipation with soiling.

Children who shower rather than bathe may miss washing the vulval area effectively; however, the most common causes of irritant contact dermatitis in children are overuse of soap and bubble bath, using shampoo in the bath, swimming in chlorinated pools and wearing occlusive clothing, often ballet and athletic gear.

Irritation from overuse of topical medications and perfumed products is very common in adults but less so in children, mainly because they are less exposed to these products. However, it is not uncommon for children with vulval symptoms to be treated with antifungal creams, which are inappropriate and often cause irritation.

Presentation

Vulval dermatitis presents with itching and a fluctuating rash, often precipitated by contact with irritants. The child's scratching behaviour is often a source of embarrassment for her parents and causes unwelcome attention at school. It is common for children with vulval itching to wake in a distressed state at night with night terrors.

Examination

Examination is often fairly unremarkable, and parents may have trouble convincing a doctor that there is anything wrong. Close inspection will reveal some erythema, scale and slight rugosity of the labia majora, and increased erythema and desquamation of the minora. The desquamation may stain the child's underwear and be misinterpreted as a vaginal discharge. If the rash is severe, it may extend to the inguinal areas and buttocks. Superinfection with *Staphylococcus aureus* may occur on the skin, but there is no vaginitis, and vaginal swabs and urine culture are negative.

Investigation

A skin swab should be performed if superinfection is suspected. Vaginal swabs are not necessary in pre-menarchal girls. A mid-stream urine sample will rule out a urinary tract infection if urinary symptoms are present.

Management

Treatment of vulval dermatitis is easy if environmental modification can be put in place.

Therefore, the first step in treating dermatitis is to modify the environment. It is preferable for girls to have a bath rather than shower. No soap or bubble bath should be used, bath oil should be used in the bath, and if the child does shower, a soap substitute should be used and the parent needs to supervise parting and rinsing of the labia. Shampoo should be rinsed out after the child gets out of the bath, or soap substitute used instead of shampoo.

If the child does gymnastics, ballet or any other physical activity that involves wearing tight Lycra clothing, if possible this should be modified so that at least during practice sessions, loose cotton clothes are worn. Even nylon tights worn as part of a school uniform may have to be discarded, and you may need to give the parents a letter to take to the school. Some recreational activities that involve contact with a saddle can also be very irritating.

When it comes to clothing, loose cotton underwear is ideal, and underpants, particularly nylon ones, should be avoided at night.

If the child is going to swimming lessons in a heated chlorinated swimming pool, keep in mind that the chlorinated water can be a powerful irritant. Applying white soft paraffin or zinc cream before swimming is helpful. The bathing costume should be removed immediately after swimming, and the skin rinsed in the shower before going home.

If the child has an incontinence problem, either with enuresis or constipation with overflow, this needs to be addressed. Parents do not always mention it out of embarrassment, and one needs to ask. Similarly, many children come to your office in underpants but are still wearing nappies at night. These should be discarded if possible. Always actively ask about this as well. Parents do not always make a connection between incontinence and vulval irritation.

The use of over-the-counter topical preparations should be enquired about. The repeated use of antifungal creams is often a cause of irritant contact dermatitis, and is particularly inappropriate in the unoestrogenised environment of childhood. Often, many household products have been used by the time the patient sees you, as well as over-the-counter medications. Again, these may not be volunteered, as the parent sees them only as an unsuccessful treatment and not a potential problem. Ask about perfumed products such as toilet paper and particularly the use of wet wipes containing methylisothiazolinone. Ask the parents to stop using all of these products. Latex can also be a problem as some parents unknowingly sensitise their children when changing their nappies while wearing latex gloves.

Specific Treatment

Most cases of vulval dermatitis will respond to hydrocortisone 1%, as long as the environmental changes have also been made. Ointment is preferable to creams, which may cause stinging. If the dermatitis is severe, a stronger non-fluorinated topical corticosteroid may be used for a week or two.

Some topical corticosteroid preparations, particularly mometasone furoate, have a tendency to sting on the vulva, and if this happens they should be avoided. Although adults can cope with this side effect, children rarely do. If a more potent corticosteroid has been used, it should be possible to reduce to hydrocortisone 1% once the rash has settled. If this is not possible, one should consider an alternative diagnosis.

Many parents are very apprehensive about using topical corticosteroids on their children, and even more so on the vulva where are they are concerned that the preparations will thin the skin. In practice, the treatment is very safe and it is wise to pre-empt any objections with strong reassurance and a warning that the pharmacist, the naturopath and well-meaning relatives may well recommend caution regarding their use.

In summary, we recommend the following:

- Avoid soap and bubble bath
- Shampoo hair in the shower not the bath
- Shower after swimming lessons and do not go home in the wet swimming costume
- Avoid perfumed wet wipes and toilet paper
- Try to dispense with night nappies or pull-ups as soon as possible
- Pay attention to constipation with overflow and dysfunctional voiding
- Avoid nylon ballet clothes and similar garments at other activities
- Ask yourself whether sporting activities that irritate the vulva (cycling, horse riding, ballet) are worth it
- Avoid nylon tights in winter
- Wear cotton underwear
- No underwear in bed at night
- Never use antifungal creams
- Use a simple non-perfumed moisturiser every day

If skin swabs show infection (usually with *S. aureus*), a course of appropriate antibiotics should be given. A finding of β-haemolytic *Streptococcus* group A requires a 10-day course of penicillin, cephalexin or, for those allergic to the former, an antibiotic such as erythromycin provided the organism is sensitive to this.

Psoriasis

Although the classic age of onset of psoriasis is early adulthood, psoriasis in children is not uncommon. If children with vulval disease are taken as a group, psoriasis is a very common cause of chronic vulval and perianal itchy rashes.

Presentation

In babies, psoriasis may present for the first time as a persistent nappy rash. The features at this age include a well-demarcated edge and involvement of the inguinal folds, but the typical scale of psoriasis is lacking under the nappy. Although it may respond to standard nappy rash treatment with hydrocortisone 1% topically, it is not unusual for the rash to be resistant to this simple treatment.

In older children, the rash is more typical of psoriasis, with an itchy, red, well-demarcated, symmetrical plaque. Again, there is no scale. The vulva, perineum, perianal area and often natal cleft may all be involved. In older children, hydrocortisone 1% is also often ineffective.

If psoriasis is confined to the vulva, it is difficult to make a definite diagnosis unless there are other diagnostic clues present. A history of cradle cap or difficult nappy rashes as a baby, nail pitting, post-auricular or scalp rashes and a family history are all helpful.

Management

Vulval psoriasis is more challenging to treat than vulval dermatitis. Although the environmental modification described above is essential, it often takes a more potent topical corticosteroid to relieve itch.

Although some cases do respond to hydrocortisone 1%, it is not uncommon for psoriasis to require stronger corticosteroids and sometimes tar creams. In this situation, referral to a dermatologist is recommended.

We usually commence a medium-potency corticosteroid ointment (preferably non-fluorinated) at night, continuing until the itch has been relieved. We then add a weak tar cream, 2% LPC (liquor picis carbonis) in a thick emollient base to be used every day, while reducing the strength of the topical corticosteroid back to hydrocortisone 1%.

The reduction in corticosteroid potency must be done gradually by initially alternating the weaker and stronger preparations, and slowly using less of the stronger one and more of the weaker one.

Most children can eventually be controlled on the weak tar cream alone. If this is not tolerated, usually because of stinging, we introduce calcipotriol 0.05% ointment for long-term control. If this is also problematic, a greasy emollient often suffices.

Lichen Sclerosus

Lichen sclerosus may start at any age, and if children with vulval disease are examined as a group, about 10% of them will have it.

Presentation

Lichen sclerosus may occur at any stage of childhood, but the average age is from 5–7 years. It is rare, and there is commonly a delay of diagnosis of at least 1 year. Girls with lichen sclerosus tend to present with more complex symptoms than adults. Itch is not always a prominent feature, and soreness, dysuria, bleeding and chronic constipation may occur. Not surprisingly, they are therefore often investigated for bowel and urinary tract abnormalities, and are sometimes referred to child protection units.

The clinical appearance is of a well-demarcated white plaque with a wrinkled surface and scattered telangiectasia. Fissuring is common, causing bleeding from time to time. The typical distribution is of a figure-of-eight plaque surrounding the vagina and anus, but any pattern on the vulva, perineum or perianal area may be seen. The vagina is not involved, and extra-genital involvement is very rare in children. Unless the labia majora are parted and a careful inspection made, it can be easy to miss this condition.

As in adults, lichen sclerosus in children can be complicated by loss of the labia minora and clitoris, which becomes buried under scar tissue.

Many children with lichen sclerosus are suspected of having been sexually abused. This relates to the unusual and unfamiliar appearance of the rash, particularly where purpura or bleeding is present. It is important for practitioners to realise that this is a skin condition. Its presence of course does not rule out abuse, but the disease itself is not a cause to suspect it.

Management

Lichen sclerosus in children is managed in exactly the same way as in adults, commencing with a super-potent topical corticosteroid and gradually reducing to the lowest strength that affects long-term control (see Chapter 4).

Parents often express fear of using such products on the vulva and are frequently cautioned by their pharmacist as well. A great deal of reassurance is required and a warning that the pharmacist may express reservations. We impress on parents the importance of effectively treating lichen sclerosus in their child to relieve symptoms and prevent loss of vulval structure.

This diagnosis can be emotionally crippling to some families who find the concept of their child having an incurable condition that will require life-long treatment of the genital area devastating. We encounter anger and denial at first in many, but most eventually come to an acceptance of the need for treatment. Some parents are squeamish about applying treatment, and negative parental attitudes are rapidly picked up by young patients. Treatment refusal follows, and many parents need much emotional support to push through the temptation to allow children to apply or dictate how often they will use their medication.

There has been controversy about whether this disease remits at puberty. Recent evidence reveals that it does not. Although symptoms may settle, silent progression of scarring and atrophy may occur, and symptom activity may recur in adult life. Adolescent girls may be too embarrassed to allow anyone to examine their genital area. It is very important, for this reason, to build up a trusting relationship with a child with lichen sclerosus, and to start warning her from about the age of 8 that when she is older she will need ongoing check-ups and treatment.

We believe that when lichen sclerosus occurs in a child, it should be treated as aggressively as in adults. Although it is relatively easy to relieve symptoms with as-needed topical corticosteroid application, the ideal outcome of management should be to preserve vulval architecture as well. Our impression, based on a detailed retrospective review of the case notes of 46 girls with pre-pubertal-onset lichen sclerosus, is that keeping the vulval skin objectively normal by using a continuous daily corticosteroid ointment will prevent burying of the clitoris and the progressive loss of the labia minora. Inadequate treatment puts the patient at risk, not only physically but also psychologically, especially in adolescence.

In addition to this, there is a worrying association (about 2–6%) with squamous cell carcinoma of the vulva in untreated lichen sclerosus in adult life. This has been reported in relatively young women who have had lichen sclerosus since childhood. Therefore, this condition should be actively managed, and follow-up should ideally be life-long. Referral to a dermatologist is recommended for initial assessment.

Birthmarks of the Vulva

Birthmarks may occur on the vulva, as on any other part of the skin, but the importance of lesions in this location is that they may be mistaken for more sinister conditions.

For example, pigmented naevi on the vulva often raise queries of melanoma, where they might be ignored elsewhere, and epidermal naevi, which are rare and therefore not familiar to general practitioners, are often mistaken for warts or recalcitrant eczema.

Haemangiomas of Infancy (Strawberry Naevi)

Haemangiomas of infancy are the most common birthmark and are found much more commonly in females. They can be located anywhere on the skin but may be located on the vulva and perianal area where they have special features:

- They are prone to ulceration, which can be so extensive that it can be difficult to tell that there was ever a birthmark present
- They may be mistaken for a sign of sexual abuse, particularly if ulcerated
- If extensive, they may be associated with abnormalities of the bladder, bowel and lumbosacral spine

The diagnostic feature of a typical haemangioma of infancy is the bright red colour, a well-defined edge and the age of onset, which is in most cases within the first 4 weeks of life. The lesions grow for a variable period, up to about 4 months of age, and then regress.

Management

In many cases, no management other than reassurance is required and, like haemangiomas elsewhere, these lesions eventually resolve. It is rare for there to be significant sequelae unless the lesions are very large or ulcerated. Large or ulcerated vulval lesions can cause severe morbidity and should be urgently referred to a dermatologist.

When ulceration occurs, it is not uncommon for a query of sexual abuse to be made. It is most important not to jump to such conclusions where there is ulceration of a haemangioma, and to seek the opinion of a dermatologist or paediatrician.

Oral propranolol has now become the treatment of choice for complex or disfiguring haemangiomas and has also been shown to effect rapid healing of ulcerated lesions. Treatment of ulceration also involves the use of ulcer dressings. Topical β-blockers have also been shown to be effective in small, flat haemangiomas, but these lesions on the vulva are usually best left in the knowledge that they will resolve spontaneously.

All complex or ulcerated haemangiomas of infancy should be referred for urgent dermatological assessment.

Pigmented Naevi

Pigmented naevi may occur on the vulva either as a congenital lesion or one that appears at any stage of childhood. The congenital lesions may be larger than late-onset ones.

It is normal for children to acquire naevi at any age on any part of the skin, and the vulva and perianal area is no exception. However, melanoma in children is rare, and there have been very few reports of childhood vulval melanoma.

The same principles apply as on any part of the skin: if a lesion has benign features, such as symmetry, even colour, growth stability and benign features on dermoscopy, it can be safely observed. Pigmented naevi of the vulva do not have any more significant malignant potential than those elsewhere and again can be safely observed. It is worth noting, however, that benign *genital* naevi can have histological features that suggest malignancy. The site of the lesion should always be specified when an excision specimen is sent for histopathological examination.

Epidermal Naevi

Epidermal naevi are quite rare and are not always present at birth. They commonly have a warty surface and may be arranged in whorls or streaks. Lesions that involve the vulva can be part of a larger one that extends to the leg and buttock.

They are sometimes very itchy and have a tendency to extend and become more raised with time, and if they become large, can interfere with function.

Because of these features, epidermal naevi can be mistaken for warts, which in turn gives rise to queries of child abuse. If they are itchy, they can be mistaken for treatment-resistant eczema or nappy rash.

It is not uncommon for epidermal naevi of the genital region to cause enough trouble to require at least partial excision. For example, a warty perianal lesion is best removed. Sometimes, recalcitrant itching is only relieved by removing the lesion.

However, if they are not causing problems, it is best just to reassure and leave them alone. They have no malignant potential.

Vulvovaginal Infections in Children

Acute Infective Vulvovaginitis

Group A β-haemolytic *Streptococcus* can cause a low-grade, persistent perianal rash (streptococcal perianal dermatitis) and also acute vulvovaginitis. This is the most common cause of acute vulvovaginitis in pre-pubertal children. It is virtually never seen in adults, although the same organism can cause vulval cellulitis at any age.

Presentation

Streptococcal vulvovaginitis presents with sudden onset of an erythematous, swollen, painful vulva and vagina, with a thin mucoid discharge.

There may have been a preceding throat infection with the same organism, or preceding perianal dermatitis. Sometimes the infection can be low grade, similar to the perianal disease, presenting as a subacute vulvitis.

It is believed that the portal of entry is the throat and that the organism reaches the vagina by haematogenous spread.

Occasionally, streptococcal genital infection may precipitate genital and/or perianal psoriasis. This is a real trap for the unwary, as it is usually interpreted as recurrent infection. A swab should always be taken if recurrence is suspected, and if it is negative, think of psoriasis.

Investigation

The infection is easily diagnosed by introital and perianal swabs. It is not necessary to insert the swab right into the vagina, which children usually find traumatic, particularly when the area is tender.

Although a differential diagnosis of acute candidiasis would be reasonable in an adult, this is not the case in children. Pre-pubertal children do not suffer from vulvovaginal candidiasis. Recurrent streptococcal infections should raise the possibility of an intra-vaginal foreign body or chronic pharyngeal carriage.

Any case of acute vulvitis in a child should suggest streptococcal vulvovaginitis, not acute candidiasis.

Management

After swabs have been taken, the child should be commenced on oral penicillin, or cephalexin if they are allergic to penicillin. Other antibiotics are used based on sensitivities. The course must run for a full 10 days or recurrence may occur. Studies have shown that also using topical mupirocin twice daily reduces the risk of recurrence.

In the past, *Haemophilus influenzae* was a frequent cause of acute paediatric vulvovaginitis. This has now become rare due to immunisation.

Staphylococcal Folliculitis and Impetigo

Staphylococcal folliculitis is common on the buttocks of children, particularly those with eczema and those who are still in night nappies. It may sometimes spread to the vulva or be found there primarily. Impetigo may also sometimes occur on the vulva and perianal area.

Presentation

The presentation is with pustules and crusted lesions, which are often more itchy and irritating rather than painful.

Investigation

The diagnosis is confirmed with a skin swab.

Management

Although impetigo usually responds quickly to a course of appropriate anti-staphylococcal antibiotics, folliculitis can be very persistent and is often better treated with topical agents such as mupirocin 2% ointment twice daily in addition for a week. Staphylococcal carriage in fomites must simultaneously be treated by adding a quarter of a cup of household bleach to the bath water and washing of clothes, sheets and towels with hot water.

Every attempt should be made to discard night nappies. If there is underlying eczema, this should be treated.

Enterobius Vermicularis (threadworm, pinworm)

Although many children with threadworm (pinworm) infestation are asymptomatic, symptoms are that of perianal and vulval itching, particularly at night. An eczematous rash may occur.

Pinworm is very well known as a cause of genital itching in children, and many children with vulval disease will already have been treated with mebendazole by their parents, prior to seeing a doctor.

Molluscum Contagiosum

These viral lesions are very common in children. The virus is spread in water. Many children are infected at public swimming pools and then transmit the infection to younger siblings with whom they share a bath. As a result, it is not uncommon for mollusca to be found on the vulva, often as part of a more generalised eruption (see Chapter 7).

Sometimes vulval mollusca can be difficult to differentiate from genital warts, and close examination with a magnifier will be needed to see the typical central core. This distinction is important, as paediatric mollusca are not sexually transmitted but paediatric genital warts may be. There are four separate mollusca genotypes, and studies have shown that the ones that cause genital lesions in adults are different to those that are usually found in children.

Management

In most cases, it is not necessary to treat vulval mollusca, as spontaneous resolution invariably occurs within 2 years. Methods used to extract the viral core from the centre, which are tolerated on less-sensitive areas, may be too painful on the vulva.

Genital Warts

Genital human papillomavirus lesions are very uncommon in children.

Genital warts should raise the question of sexual abuse, and many experts recommend that a consultation with a child protection unit should be arranged. This is invariably traumatic for the family and unfortunately it is often difficult even for experts to draw a firm conclusion. Unless either the child or a parent discloses that sexual abuse has occurred, no action can be taken unless sexually transmissible infection screening reveals an infection that is definitively sexually transmitted, for example gonorrhoea.

There are many articles in the medical literature that state that there are many ways genital warts can be acquired in children other than sexually, but we do not see the logic in asserting this in children, while assuming that they are invariably sexually acquired in adults (see Chapter 7). Unfortunately, this remains an area of controversy. There is probably truth in the contention that not all genital warts in children are sexually acquired, but convincing research to support how common this is relative to sexual transmission is lacking.

Presentation

Genital warts typically have a filiform appearance and may involve the vulva, vaginal introitus and perianal area.

These lesions are usually small but can occasionally become large enough to interfere with toilet routines.

Management

Imiquimod and podophyllotoxin may be safely used in children and are preferable as first-line treatments to painful modalities such as cryotherapy or cautery, which require a general anaesthetic.

In children with very extensive perianal warts, surgical debulking may be required before this treatment is commenced.

Genital Herpes

Herpetic lesions of the vulval area are very uncommon in children. In infancy, herpes can be acquired at birth from a mother with genital herpes, or inoculated from an adult with a herpetic lesion on the mouth or finger.

Children with severe atopic eczema are also prone to unusual herpetic infections in unusual locations, and this may involve the genital area.

Presentation

The clinical findings are the same as in adults: painful vesicles that rapidly erode and ulcerate, associated with lymphadenopathy. There is sometimes some degree of oedema of the labia.

Investigation

The finding of a primary attack of genital herpes in an older child should be confirmed by PCR, and should raise the possibility of sexual abuse. The subject of whether a child with herpes of the genital region has been sexually abused is even more difficult than with genital warts because there are a number of innocent ways that a child might acquire genital herpes.

The differential diagnosis of herpes includes two very uncommon conditions: vulval aphthous ulcers and vulval bullous pemphigoid (see Chapter 5). Both present with painful ulcerating lesions, and it is not surprising that they are often mistaken for herpes. However, herpes PCR is negative, and sexual abuse should not be suspected on the grounds of these lesions.

Management

Genital herpes in children is treated in the same way as in adults using oral antiviral medication.

Fungal Infections

Tinea is a common cause of groin rashes in men and sometimes causes vulval rashes in women, but it is rarely found on the vulva in children. When it does occur, it hardly ever has typical features, and is often the result of treatment with topical corticosteroids. It may be more common than one would think, as so many cases of vulval rashes are treated with imidazole creams, which fortuitously also treat tinea.

Presentation

In cases where no antifungal has been used, tinea of the vulva or under the nappy in a baby presents as a dermatitic rash that does not respond to topical corticosteroid treatment.

Investigation

The diagnosis requires a high index of suspicion but once suspected is easily confirmed by a skin scraping.

Candidiasis, on the other hand, does not occur in children out of nappies. In adults with chronic vulval symptoms, about 15% have candidiasis, but this oestrogen-dependent condition is not seen after infancy in children with normal immune systems.

This is an important point, as it is common for children with skin diseases such as dermatitis and psoriasis to be diagnosed with thrush and treated with antifungal creams, which may cause irritation, particularly if dermatitis is present.

Anatomical Abnormalities

Fusion of the Labia Minora

Fusion of the labia is sometimes seen in young children, usually 3 years of age and under. It is not seen in adults, unless they have scarring skin diseases such as lichen sclerosus or lichen planus.

Fusion of the labia is not a malformation and is acquired. It may appear from birth.

Presentation

It is not clear why this happens to some children, but many do have an underlying dermatitis. Not all are symptomatic, but some experience soreness or itching. Urine can pool behind the fusion causing irritating maceration as well as slow urination. Urinary tract infections are, however, rarely a complicating factor.

The labia minora or majora are agglutinated to a variable degree from the tip of the clitoris to the posterior fourchette. This may result in an abnormal-looking vulva with no apparent vaginal opening.

Investigation

Fusion of the labia is important in the differential diagnosis of ambiguous genitalia and an imperforate hymen, and a specialist opinion should be sought if there is any doubt.

Management

This is the only condition where oestrogen cream is the treatment of choice in a pre-pubertal child. The cream need only be applied once a day, and the fusion usually resolves over a 2–6-week period. Once the fusion has separated, ongoing treatment with soap avoidance, topical lubricants and hydrocortisone 1% is recommended.

The fusion may reform and have to be retreated from time to time. This can be a problem as oestrogen creams are irritating in children and make cooperation difficult.

Very occasionally, a minor surgical procedure to separate the agglutinated labia may be required. The condition tends to resolve spontaneously in older children.

Pyramidal Perineal Protrusion

Although this has only recently been labelled as an entity in the medical literature, it is probably not rare. It is noticed in infancy as an asymptomatic soft protrusion of the median raphe in girls. The overlying skin is normal.

This condition can be confused with genital warts.

The aetiology of this condition is unknown and there are no consistent associations with other conditions. It is not consistently the result of constipation and it resolves spontaneously.

No treatment is required.

Foreign Bodies

Although intra-vaginal foreign bodies are often mentioned as a cause of vulval disease in the medical literature, in fact they are not a common event. The foreign material is usually a fragment of toilet paper or fluff. Small toys are less common.

The child presents with a persistent purulent discharge heavy enough to cause maceration of the vulval skin. Swabs show recurrent bacterial infection, which responds to courses of antibiotics but rapidly recurs.

The child will require examination under anaesthesia and saline lavage. Often, there is very little to be seen on lavage, and it is likely that small fragments can cause this clinical presentation.

Labia Minora in Children and Adolescents: Size and Labial Asymmetry – What Is Normal?

Pre-pubertal children normally have very small labia minora; however, around puberty, they enlarge to the normal structures found in adults.

There is a very large variation in the size and bulk of labia minora. Rarely, they are congenitally absent, but the vast majority of women have them and their absence during reproductive life is not normal.

In some girls, the labia grow asymmetrically, with one side growing first and the other catching up later. It is not uncommon for some minor degree of asymmetry to be present, but in some individuals this is so marked that it becomes a source of embarrassment – particularly in adolescence.

Very large labia minora can also occur bilaterally and can become not only embarrassing but uncomfortable. As a result, patients may request surgical correction. This is called 'reduction labioplasty'.

Labioplasty is becoming more and more widely requested. It is very important to understand the motivation of the patient: there is a difference between trimming large labia that are producing genuine discomfort and reducing normal labia for purely cosmetic reasons. Moreover, the complaint of large, uncomfortable labia may in fact be a presentation of a skin disease such as psoriasis.

It is not our place to pass judgement on those who perform this procedure, however, except to point out that it is not without risk, and patients should be adequately assessed, and fully informed, before proceeding.

Psychological Aspects of Vulval Problems in Children

In adults with vulval pain (and less commonly itch), there is a small but significant group who present with symptoms but with no apparent abnormality. Although some are malingering or somaticising, there are many more who have a genuine complaint of neuropathy or referred pain.

When a child presents with symptoms but a normal-appearing vulva, even after close examination when symptoms are maximal, it is unlikely that there is any physical cause. It is always worth checking for a scoliosis and obtaining a physiotherapy assessment if the child's complaints raise a suspicion of neuropathy. However, neuropathic pain in pre-pubertal girls is rare.

A common scenario is the child who presents because of a greenish discharge noticed as staining of the underwear. There are no symptoms other than the discharge, and swabs and urine culture are normal. This situation is a normal variant.

A somewhat less innocent situation is a child who constantly complains of vulval discomfort in the absence of findings and without any observable sign of being in pain. Children rapidly realise that complaining of genital pain, particularly at school or in public, attracts adult attention and is a source of embarrassment for their parents.

They may even find that worried teachers rapidly send them home from school, and distraught parents are then summoned to answer sexual abuse allegations.

In other words, havoc can be created, not only for the parents but also for the unwary clinician!

Children who do this have no idea how much distress they are causing but know that it is an effective attention-seeking device. The best way to deal with it is usually to withdraw the attention, but occasionally psychiatric help is needed.

Sometimes, a child's complaint of vulval pain may be a smokescreen for her habit of masturbation. This can happen if her parents are shocked by this behaviour. It is then necessary to help the parents come to terms with the normality of the child's actions.

In most of these cases, non-intervention, reassurance and not giving in to attention-getting behaviour are the best treatment.

Vulval Disease and Sexual Abuse: What Should You Do?

Most parents of a child with a vulval condition of any sort will have considered the possibility of sexual abuse, even though they often do not tend to voice it, particularly at the first visit. It is reasonable for them to do so.

Child sexual abuse and paedophilia have received enormous publicity in the lay press; however, there are never any details of what physical evidence there might be in an abused child, and this is therefore left up to the imagination.

Professionals who deal with children are also made very aware of child abuse as an issue because of legal requirements to reveal criminal records as a condition of employment. It is therefore common for carers and teachers to have these concerns about children who scratch the vulval area constantly or complain of vulval pain. Parents who suspect abuse in a child with a vulval condition may blame persons who care for the child in their absence.

Doctors in many countries are required by law to report any suspected case of sexual abuse, and when a general practitioner is faced with a vulval condition, they too may consider sexual abuse. However, this presents them with a very difficult problem. Reporting the patient may well ruin the doctor–patient relationship, and may result in an unnecessary, distressing invasion of privacy if they are proven to be incorrect. A strong suspicion of sexual abuse may by law prompt a report, but often it is by no means easy to make this decision.

The vulval conditions that should prompt doctors to consider sexual abuse are not the dermatoses such as psoriasis and lichen sclerosus but the infectious diseases that may be sexually transmissible.

The situation, however, is far from straightforward. When it comes to genital warts, there are enough articles in the medical literature stating that these lesions in children are rarely sexually transmissible to make this an area of ongoing controversy. It is also genuinely possible that genital herpes in a child can be the result of non-sexual transmission, particularly if there is an underlying condition such as eczema.

Even in expert hands, diagnosing sexual abuse is very difficult and impossible to prove without a disclosure from the child or a relative. Many cases remain unresolved, even after investigation and interview in the child protection unit setting.

Numerous retrospective studies confirm that about 20% of adult women were in some way sexually abused as children. This does not necessarily mean sexual intercourse, however; all forms of unwelcome and inappropriate sexual contact in childhood can have devastating long-term psychological implications.

Perpetrators of sexual abuse are usually well known to the child, often relatives and close family friends who blackmail them into remaining silent. Child sexual abuse within the family is society's well-kept secret. It is almost never spoken of, and the likelihood of obtaining a disclosure from any family member or the child is remote. Without disclosure, it is very difficult for any further action to be taken. Although institutionalised sexual abuse is now receiving much attention, studies show that child sexual abuse within the family unit and close acquaintances is common. This is very difficult to address. One can only hope that the experience of being questioned by a health professional will encourage the family to act of their own accord.

Most children who have been sexually abused do not have any physical signs, because trauma such as bruises resolves quickly, and abusive behaviour often does not involve attempts at penetration.

The presence of a rash such as eczema, psoriasis or lichen sclerosus should not raise queries of abuse. The child may well have been abused, but the rash in itself is not evidence, and there would have to be other reasons to suspect it.

In cases where the child has an infection that may have been acquired sexually such as genital warts or genital herpes, the issue of sexual abuse should be raised, and if there is no obvious explanation of non-sexual transmission, there are grounds to report.

Where there is a suspicion of sexual abuse, consultation with a child protection unit is the best first step. Child protection units are found in tertiary referral children's hospitals. We recommend you call a child protection unit and speak to a paediatrician working there. This usually provides clarity about what to do next. If you have referred your patient and the family refuses to be assessed or does not attend their appointment, consult the child protection unit regarding your legal obligations.

When a child presents with a vulval rash, parents often have unvoiced concerns about sexual abuse, so it is worth discussing this. They will usually be greatly relieved that their child simply has a skin problem.

The medical literature contains many cases where skin conditions have been mistaken for sexual abuse, and this includes lichen sclerosus, ulcerated haemangiomas and rare skin conditions such as bullous pemphigoid, which may cause genital ulcers.

It is important to understand that lay people may attribute almost any vulval condition to sexual abuse. Although the presence of a skin condition does not rule it out, there would have to be other grounds to suspect it such as household composition, parental concerns, the presence of sexually acquired infections and behavioural abnormalities in the child.

General Management Principles

Diagnosing the Problem

Keep in mind that most cases of vulval itching in pre-pubertal girls will be due to dermatitis, either atopic or the result of irritation from clothing or applied substances. Also remember that there is often a much greater emotional overlay attached to any condition of the genital area than in other parts of the skin. As a result, the degree of distress experienced by the parents and sometimes the child may be out of proportion to the actual problem.

There is still a tendency for vulval disease to be poorly understood, and it is not uncommon for patients to visit many doctors without receiving what they consider a satisfactory explanation, and effective treatment. As a result, parents are often angry and frustrated. This can make history taking difficult, and may leave the doctor wondering why the emotional reaction is so intense when there is so little to see.

Where examination reveals little more than a dermatitic poorly defined rash, it is likely that the child does have dermatitis. Look carefully, as the signs can be subtle. Avoid dismissing the examination as normal if there are significant symptoms. It is reasonable to take a vulval swab to rule out superinfection.

Urinary frequency or dysuria can sometimes result from dermatitic irritation of the urethral meatus. A urine culture may be necessary to exclude infection but is usually normal.

When the rash is erythematous but well defined, and particularly when there is perianal involvement, look for other signs of psoriasis and enquire about a family history.

A white, well-defined eruption should suggest lichen sclerosus. These cases should be referred to a dermatologist.

If pustules or weeping areas are present, always perform a skin swab. If herpes simplex is suspected, viral swabs for PCR are indicated. For a vaginal discharge, use a swab moistened with saline to gently sample from the introitus. Vaginal swabs are not necessary, and will cause distress to the child and parent. A skin scraping is indicated where a dermatitic rash has been persistent despite treatment.

Check that the child has been treated for possible pinworm infestation.

Psychological Management

Much stronger reassurance is often required when skin disease affects the vulva than when it is found on other skin areas. Always enquire about fears of sexually transmissible disease and child abuse.

It is best to be matter of fact and help the parents to understand that the vulva is simply part of the skin. Inform them that children rapidly pick up their anxieties, and that an intelligent child may capitalise on this with attention-seeking or school-avoidance behaviour.

You should refer in the following situations (Table 9.1):

- The diagnosis is uncertain, or there is an apparent non-response to treatment. In practice, non-response is often a result of non-compliance, which is in turn the result of anxiety about the condition. Extra reassurance may be required.
- In the case of proven infection that is recurrent. There may be an underlying abnormality causing the recurrence, such as a foreign body.
- The child with an ulcerating lesion. Most ulcers are not traumatic but pathological, with aphthous ulcers being the most common.
- You suspect the child has lichen sclerosus.
- The child has a labial fusion.
- There is a concern about sexual abuse.

Table 9.1 Causes of vulval disease in children

Red itchy rash	Eczema
	Psoriasis
	Tinea
	Folliculitis
	Allergic contact dermatitis
	Vaginal foreign body with persistent discharge
White rash	Lichen sclerosus
Blisters, erosions or ulcers	Impetigo
	Herpes simplex
	Herpes zoster
	Varicella
	Aphthous ulcers
	Bullous pemphigoid
	Erythema multiforme
Acute vulvovaginitis	Group A β-haemolytic streptococcal vulvovaginitis
	Fixed drug eruption
	Erythema multiforme
Lesions	Molluscum contagiosum
	Human papillomavirus
	Pyramidal perineal protrusion
	Birthmarks
	Haemangiomas
Normal-appearing vulva	Subacute vulvitis
	Pinworm
	Attention-getting behaviour

Further Reading

Ellis, E. and Fischer, G. (2015). Prepubertal onset vulvar lichen sclerosus: the importance of maintenance therapy in long-term outcomes. *Pediatric Dermatology*, **32**, 461–7.

Fischer, G. (2010). Chronic vulvitis in pre-pubertal girls. *Australasian Journal of Dermatology*, **51**, 118–23.

Fischer, G. O. (2001). Vulval disease in pre-pubertal girls. *Australasian Journal of Dermatology*, **42**, 225–36.

Fischer, G. O. (2011). Genital disease in children. Part 26 Ch 151 In Irvine, A. D., Hoeger, P. H. and Yan, A. C., eds, *Harper's Textbook of Pediatric Dermatology*, 3rd edn. Hoboken, NJ: Wiley-Blackwell.

Fischer, G. O. and Rogers, M. (2000). Vulvar diseases in children. A clinical audit of 130 cases. *Pediatric Dermatology*, **17**, 1–6.

Hong, E. and Fischer, G. (2012). Propranolol for recalcitrant ulcerated haemangioma of infancy. *Pediatric Dermatology*, **29**, 64–7.

Jayasinghe, Y. and Garland, S. M. (2006). Genital warts in children: what do they mean? *Archives of Disease in Childhood*, **91**, 696–700.

Reed, B. D. and Cantor, L. E. (2008). Vulvodynia in preadolescent girls. *Journal of Lower Genital Tract Disease*, **12**, 257–61.

Smith, S. and Fischer, G. (2009). Lichen sclerosus in girls: a review. *Australasian Journal of Dermatology*, **50**, 243–8.

Chapter 10

Myths and Pearls

Myths ...

... about Thrush

Most Itchy Vulval Conditions Are Due to Thrush

Acute thrush is very common. Everyone has heard of it and it even features in television advertisements for antifungal treatments. However, although it is usually the first thought of patients, pharmacists and even doctors, there are many conditions other than thrush that can cause vulval problems, particularly when it comes to chronic conditions.

For a patient with a long-standing chronic vulvitis, chronic thrush represents the minority (about 20%) of all cases. Many patients tell us that their doctor prescribed antifungal medication without either examining them or taking a vaginal swab.

While it may be acceptable to do this on the first presentation, it is not best practice to use multiple courses of antifungals without confirmation of candidiasis on a vaginal swab. Unfortunately, when a patient has been given multiple courses of topical and/or oral antifungal agents, the false-negative rate of such swabs is very high. Particularly for patients with chronic vulvovaginal candidiasis, the length of time that the patient needs to be withdrawn from such agents before their swab can be recorded as positive again can be very prolonged. We therefore strongly recommend that patients always have a vaginal swab before any treatment is commenced.

Pre-pubertal Children Suffer from Vaginal Thrush

This is completely untrue. Healthy pre-pubertal children who are out of nappies do not suffer from thrush. Thrush may be seen in the setting of chronic maceration (incontinence), immunodeficiency and diabetes.

Thrush requires an oestrogenised environment and is therefore not seen before puberty. In Australia, the only infective vaginitis we see with any frequency is due to group A *Streptococcus*.

A child with an itchy vulvitis should never be assumed to have thrush, and antifungal creams will not be effective.

Post-menopausal Women Can Suffer from Vaginal Thrush

Adequate oestrogen levels are necessary for a woman to acquire a vaginal candidiasis infection and therefore thrush is not seen in post-menopausal women.

The only exceptions to this rule are:

- Women using hormone-replacement therapy or vaginal oestrogens
- Women with diabetes
- Women with an underlying vulval skin disease such as lichen sclerosus
- Women who have overused topical steroids on the vulva
- Women who are immunosuppressed

Probiotics and the Anti-*Candida* Diet Are the 'Natural' Answer for Thrush

This is a very popular concept. The anti-*Candida* diet is very difficult to comply with and probiotics are expensive. The patients we see have usually tried them without success.

There is no clinical trial that shows that either of these methods is effective. Nevertheless, many patients want to explore 'natural' therapy and we respect their right to do so. We are happy to see them again for medical treatment if they have not improved.

Long-term Oral Antifungal Drugs Will Harm Your Liver

The first oral anti-*Candida* medication available was ketoconazole. This medication did have a real risk of drug-induced hepatitis, in the order of 10%. As a result, all patients on ketoconazole had to have regular liver function tests.

The more recent oral anti-*Candida* medications recommended in this book, itraconazole and fluconazole, do not have a high risk of liver damage, and our experience with both of these drugs, even when taken long term, is that they have an excellent safety record, similar to the long-term use of antiviral medication.

It is not logical that there is a high rate of acceptance of long-term antiviral medication to control recurrent genital herpes and yet a fear of using oral azoles long-term to control chronic candidiasis.

The main disadvantage of these medications is not liver damage but cost and possible drug interactions, particularly with lipid-lowering statin medication.

Chronic Thrush Can Be Managed by a Weekly Dose of Fluconazole

This is a notion that is widely held because there have been publications that recommend it. Furthermore, it is convenient, as these single doses of fluconazole can be purchased over the counter. It does work for some patients. Nevertheless, we see many failures from this regimen.

We believe that the best way to bring chronic thrush under control initially is with daily oral antifungal treatment. Intermittent regimens are appropriate once control has been achieved, but not before.

…about Oestrogen

If the Antifungal Has Not Worked, Try a Topical Oestrogen

We see many patients who have been prescribed an antifungal cream and when this did not work, a topical oestrogen, both without benefit.

There is only one condition in adults for whom topical oestrogen will have any benefit: oestrogen deficiency. This pertains only to post-menopausal and lactating women.

Topical oestrogens are rapidly effective. If they have not worked in 6 weeks, look for another diagnosis and cease this treatment.

In children, there is only one appropriate condition that should be treated with topical oestrogen and that is fusion of the labia. It is completely inappropriate to use topical oestrogen in a child in any other situation. It will be ineffective and is very likely to sting.

Hormone-replacement Therapy Does Not Cause Thrush or Allergies

This is also completely untrue. We see post-menopausal women who have intractable thrush until they cease their hormone-replacement therapy. In a post-menopausal woman on hormone-replacement therapy who has thrush, it should be assumed that this is responsible.

Furthermore, the thrush will not be easily controllable until the hormone-replacement therapy is temporarily ceased while it is treated with antifungal agents.

With respect to allergies, vaginal creams and pessaries not uncommonly cause an irritant vaginitis, which is reversible when the treatment is ceased.

Many allergic skin reactions to systemic hormone-replacement therapy have been described, and we sometimes see women with similar vaginal allergic reactions to it.

…about Lichen Sclerosus

Lichen Sclerosus Can Be Managed Long Term with Once- or Twice-weekly Treatment

There have been many reviews of lichen sclerosus that authoritatively state this. These opinion pieces have been based on a small number of older, short-term research studies, which claimed that it was possible to control the condition using twice-weekly ultra-potent topical corticosteroid. These have now been superseded by our prospective study of lichen sclerosus, which confirms that there is no 'one size fits all' treatment for lichen sclerosus. We recommend that treatment be tailored to the individual patient for best results and high levels of long-term control (see Chapter 4).

Lichen Sclerosus Does Not Require Follow-Up

This myth has arisen because active lichen sclerosus may be asymptomatic for long periods of time. Lichen sclerosus probably remits only occasionally.

The majority of patients, if withdrawn from therapy, will eventually have a recurrence of their symptoms, and by the time this happens, there will frequently be more irreversible damage.

Careful follow-up of lichen sclerosus is important in order to:

- Monitor for cancer
- Adjust treatment
- Check for side effects of treatment
- Make sure scarring is not interfering with the patient's life
- Encourage ongoing compliance
- Empower your patient to resist the many influences that tell her that long-term use of topical corticosteroids is dangerous

If a patient's topical steroid requirements decrease so that they are using only hydrocortisone 1%, a trial of cessation of therapy is reasonable. Try to impress on your patient that, even if they may remain asymptomatic, the disease may reactivate.

If possible, patients should not be entirely discharged from care until they have been objectively disease free for a year. About half of our patients eventually are lost to follow-up. There are probably many reasons for this. We hope their GPs or other doctors are successfully managing them or that they have gone into remission.

…about Topical Corticosteroids

Topical corticosteroid phobia is at epidemic proportions. Unfortunately, much of this fear derives from the incorrect attribution of systemic corticosteroid side effects to the topical agents.

The words 'use sparingly' that are invariably placed on labels by pharmacists are frightening to patients who wonder why this is emphasised. The internet has also sensationalised the dangers of these medications, and the popular push for all things 'natural' has demonised them as truly hazardous.

The fact is that topical corticosteroids have been in use for over 60 years, we have extensive knowledge of them and, if used correctly, they are very safe.

The notion that skin will be somehow 'thinned' by topical corticosteroids is the most pervading fear. (Most patients when asked what they think this means are not really sure.) The super-potent corticosteroid clobetasol propionate may do this with prolonged use. This medication has, unfortunately, become synonymous with treatment of vulval disease as it was the first topical corticosteroid reported to be effective for lichen sclerosus. As a result, most subsequent trials employed it, in our opinion unnecessarily. Although it is useful for severe cases of lichen sclerosus and for lichen planus, it is rarely required to treat other vulval conditions, and weaker topical corticosteroids do not share its hazards.

On the vulva, 'thin skin' would mean visible veins, striae and fragility so that the skin would tear during intercourse. In fact, we do not see this very often in our practices.

In general, in the genital area, the use of a weak topical corticosteroid such as hydrocortisone 1% is very safe, even long term. Stronger steroids may be used when needed, particularly in lichen sclerosus.

In reality, the main side effect we see from topical corticosteroid use is redness associated with a burning sensation. This reverses when a lower-potency steroid is used. In some lichen sclerosus patients who have high steroid requirements, candidiasis can supervene; however, this is surprisingly rare.

...that Psoriasis Can Be Cured

Psoriasis is a chronic endogenous dermatosis for which there is most certainly no cure. Psoriasis may unpredictably go into remission for long periods of time. However, there is always the risk that it will reactivate, particularly at times of emotional stress.

Always be very honest about the prognosis in patients with psoriasis. Even though a cure is not possible, this disease can be controlled, although this can be more difficult for some patients than for others. It is very unusual to find a patient with vulval psoriasis who is unable to control her condition with regular topical treatment.

Many cases of psoriasis are mistakenly thought to be an allergic or irritant dermatitis, which potentially *can* be cured (see Chapter 2). If such a patient re-presents when you thought they should have been cured, you may be dealing with psoriasis.

...that Vulval Disease Is Primarily Gynaecological

Vulval problems do not come under any one specialty. Gynaecology plays a role, but the dominant specialty involved is dermatology. However, pain management, neurology, gynaecological oncology, sexual health, physiotherapy and psychotherapy may all be important in certain patients.

Being a 'vulvologist' involves some knowledge of all these areas, although no one person can have complete expertise. This is what makes vulval disease a truly multidisciplinary area.

The vulva is part of the skin with its own unique features. The outside of the vulva has much in common with the axilla because of the presence of hair and apocrine sweat glands, the lack of sun exposure and its tendency to maceration.

The inner vulva has a great deal in common with the inside of the mouth. The lining of the vagina is keratinising mucosa with mucous glands and sebaceous glands.

Of the diseases that involve the vulva, the majority of those that have objective signs are skin diseases and therefore come under the umbrella of dermatology. Diseases that involve the vagina such as lichen planus and autoimmune blistering diseases are also dermatological conditions, as are allergic reactions to suppositories, condoms and semen.

Gynaecological conditions that cause vulval disease are vaginitis due to infections such as chronic thrush and non-infective causes such as desquamative inflammatory vulvovaginitis.

Gynaecology is of great importance in the field of vulval cancer, vulval conditions requiring surgery and where hormonal influences play a role in vulval disease. This includes oestrogen-hypersensitivity vulvitis, atrophic vulvovaginitis and post-menopausal women with vulval conditions where there are issues related to hormone-replacement therapy.

…that When All Else Has Failed, Take a Biopsy

Biopsies should be undertaken only if there is an objective abnormality.

There are many reasons for treatment failure. These include:

- Non-compliance, often due to corticosteroid phobia
- The patient's own well-meaning hygiene habits
- Sporting activities that irritate the skin
- Undiagnosed infection
- Allergy to a medication, condom, semen or over-the-counter preparations
- Incorrect diagnosis, especially of musculoskeletal and neuropathic pain
- Psychological problems

None of these problems will be elucidated by a biopsy. If the vulva looks normal, the biopsy will be normal as well. Take another history and keep the above in mind.

…that Vulvodynia Is a Disease

Vulvodynia is a symptom, not a disease. The word literally means vulval pain. The International Society for the Study of Vulvar Disease (ISSVD) definition includes rawness, irritation and burning.

Vulvodynia is as much a disease as 'headache'. It is a non-specific term and is a symptom of virtually every disease that affects the vulva.

…that Women Who Complain of Chronic Vulval Symptoms Often Have a Psychiatric Disorder

When we were trainee specialists in the 1980s, this was a very common belief. Our subsequent experience, however, has been that vulval symptoms are no more due primarily to psychiatric disease than any other set of symptoms. In the last few years, as the field of vulval disease is becoming recognised and good-quality research is appearing, we have seen this attitude become much less prevalent.

There is no doubt that women with chronic vulval symptoms have high rates of anxiety, depression and sexual disorders, but our opinion is that these are usually secondary to the physical vulval disease.

Pelvic floor muscle spasm does appear to be triggered in some cases by psychological issues, but even in this situation, the cure relies heavily on physiotherapy rather than psychotherapy.

Many women do feel a sense of relief that their vulval disease has legitimised their pre-existing reduction in sexual interest, and some of them refuse to have sexual intercourse with their partners again, even when they have objectively recovered. This may be manipulative or even dishonest but is a life choice, not madness.

…that There Is Such a Thing as an Ideal Vulva

The vulva is a bit like the face: there are as many different vulvas as there are faces. This is true of size, shape, colour and amount and texture of genital hair. When a patient, particularly an adolescent, comes to see you worried about the appearance of their labia, you have to be able to tell her confidently that everyone is different and there is no such thing as 'normal'. We, like many other health professionals, are not in favour of the rise of cosmetic labioplasty. Any patient has the right to have cosmetic surgery, despite the expense and risks, but we do not believe that having smaller labia minora will enhance a woman's sexual pleasure. We are also disturbed by the way that these women have been convinced that they are 'abnormal'. An excellent website for your patients to have a look at is http://www.labialibrary.org.au.

Pearls

Environmental Modification Is Key, no Matter What Your Patient Suffers From

Every vulval condition will benefit from environmental modification. The minimum each patient should be doing includes:

- Avoiding all contact with soap
- Wearing cotton underwear
- Using tampons rather than pads
- Never wearing liners
- Never wearing G-strings
- Using a clipper or having laser treatment for hair removal instead of shaving or waxing
- Wearing underwear and pants that are loose enough to be comfortable
- Not wearing Lycra at the gym
- Avoiding sporting activities that cause heavy sweating and overheating
- Using a non-irritating lubricant such as vegetable oil
- Avoiding perfumed feminine hygiene products and wet wipes
- Abstaining from sex if it hurts

Realise that Anything Genital Is Highly Emotionally Charged

A patient with a genital rash will always attach a great deal more anxiety and significance to it than if the same skin disease occurred on another part of the skin.

Patients may also have anxieties about sex that cause anxiety about any genital rash.

Always Ask about Sexual Functioning, Even if Your Patient Does Not Mention It

Many patients are too embarrassed to talk about pain with intercourse. Even when this is their main complaint they will often open their conversation with you in a very roundabout way and it is not until you specifically ask if this is their main problem that they admit to it.

There is often a high degree of shame associated with not being able to function 'normally'. The popular press virtually never depicts sex as unpleasant and patients' expectations reflect this.

Ask about Faecal Incontinence

Faecal staining of underwear is not uncommon in older women, but such women will rarely volunteer this important information because of embarrassment. It is often caused by genuine faecal incontinence but can be caused by inadequate cleaning due to obesity, arthritis or poor eyesight.

We see many older women whose vulval problems, which were previously thought intractable, become much easier to manage when their rectal problems improved. Even though faecal incontinence may not be curable in many cases, there are simple measures that will help: the application of petroleum jelly over the anus before each bowel motion, and using a hairdryer on the cool setting to properly dry genital skin.

Reassure Your Patient That it is not Cancer or a Sexually Transmissible Infection

The two things that patients fear and are often too embarrassed to mention are sexually transmissible infections and cancer. Always ask if they are concerned about either or both of these issues. Keep in mind also that repeated studies tell us that 20% of women were in some way sexually abused as children. They may have suppressed this or have kept it a secret all their lives.

Any genital problem will make them wonder if there is a connection between what is going on now and what may have happened to them in the past. However, most genital diseases fall well outside this narrow range of frightening possibilities and are benign skin diseases.

Emphasising that their disease is not a sexually transmissible infection or a cancer is very reassuring. Keep in mind, however, that your patient may be so anxious that very little of what you say has been understood in the way you hoped it would be. Information sheets that can be read later are very helpful.

Reassure Your Patient She cannot 'Give This' to Her Partner

Again, even when you think you have fully explained a benign skin disorder to your patient, you cannot assume that they will understand that it is not transmissible.

The question 'Can I give this to my partner?' after you have just spent 10 minutes explaining psoriasis may seem ridiculous to you, but many lay people have trouble grasping the difference between something infective and something endogenous.

Most patients assume that skin disorders are mostly infective and that the vulva is no exception.

With a Child, Always Ask the Parents Whether They Are Worried about Sexual Abuse, Even When They Have not Mentioned It

When a child presents with a genital problem the issue of sexual abuse is often on parents' minds, even if they do not immediately voice it. Again, ask specifically.

Although skin disease does not rule out sexual abuse, neither is it a reason alone to suspect it.

This is a very different situation, however, to possible sexually transmissible infections such as genital warts or genital herpes. Here, it is essential to consider the possibility of child abuse.

The medical literature on sexual abuse tells us that perpetrators are usually known and trusted by the child, so they are frequently family members.

This is unbearably painful for the parents of the child, and it is only natural that if a child goes to any form of childcare, parents will be directing their suspicions there, rather than at the immediate family. This sometimes has disastrous consequences for innocent child care workers.

Make Sure She Has Something to Read That Is Factual and Accurate

Although it is not universal, most patients will go straight to their computer when they get home and look up their condition and its treatment on the internet. Some do this more than others, but there are very few who will not do some research of their own.

When it comes to vulval disease, the internet is full of frightening, complex and sometimes inaccurate data. It is helpful to have information sheets and to direct patients to websites that are factual.

The following websites contain good, factual information:

- Care Down There: http://www.caredownthere.com.au
- British Society for the Study of Vulval Disease: http://www.bssvd.org
- International Society for the Study of Vulvar Disease: http://www.issvd.org

How to Do a Vulval Biopsy

We perform this minor procedure in the rooms and it is usually kinder to do it at the first consultation if possible. Sending patients home with an appointment to come back for the biopsy at a later date just gives them more time to worry about it.

Remember that in order to make a histopathological diagnosis of a skin condition, a piece of tissue about 3 mm in diameter to a depth of about 3 mm is all that is required.

To anaesthetise the skin, we inject about 0.1 ml of 1–2% xylocaine with adrenalin directly under the area to be biopsied, intradermally. If your patient is very apprehensive, topical anaesthetic cream may be applied before injecting. This should be left on for at least 20 minutes to be effective.

We do not use an antiseptic preparation on mucosa, as they are all likely to sting and irritate. On hair-bearing skin, any preparation such as povidone iodine or chlorhexidine may be used.

Before performing the biopsy, test with a sharp instrument to make sure the area is numb. There are two very easy and quick procedures:

1. Snip: suitable for lesions on the soft mucosal surface. Simply pinch up a small fold of skin with fine Adson forceps and then cut a small ellipse under the forceps.
2. Punch biopsy: suitable for lesions on hair-bearing skin or for a firm lesion on the mucosal surface that is difficult to grasp with forceps. Use a round 3 mm punch, twiddle while applying pressure to the lesion to a depth of 3 mm and then withdraw the punch. The core of skin is then lifted up with forceps and snipped off with fine scissors.

It is not necessary to suture biopsies of 3 mm or smaller. Haemostasis is achieved with a haemostatic agent such as silver nitrate. We give the patient a panty liner to wear home in case of minor bleeding. No specific aftercare is required, but the patient should not have intercourse for a week or until the wound has healed.

There are some situations where it is best to formally excise a lesion in its entirety. In this situation, traditional surgical techniques with scalpel excision and a suture are used. It is usually not appropriate to attempt such a procedure in the office unless you are experienced in skin surgery.

How to Use Topical Corticosteroids on the Vulva

Topical corticosteroids are very safe if used appropriately and are very unlikely to have any side effects. It is normal to use them on the vulva to treat inflammatory skin disease.

For acute management of eczema or psoriasis, we use either hydrocortisone 1% for mild inflammation or a medium-potency ointment for more severe inflammation.

These will need to be continued for 1 month or longer, depending on whether the particular condition is self-limiting or chronic. Any topical corticosteroid stronger than these preparations is generally not indicated.

The most frequent condition that requires long-term topical corticosteroids is lichen sclerosus.

Available corticosteroid preparations vary widely from country to country. Long-term corticosteroid use for lichen sclerosus is most safely achieved with a moderate-strength non-fluorinated preparation. If this is not available, then a combination of weak and moderate to strong agents, used on alternate nights, usually provides an adequate alternative. Clinicians should familiarise themselves with which preparations (weak, moderate and strong) are available in their country.

In order to use topical corticosteroids safely, the following should be done:

- Titrate the strength of the preparation to match the severity of the disease and reduce to a lower strength as soon as there is an adequate response.
- Use moderate to weak preparations for maintenance treatment.
- Do not ever leave a patient on a potent topical corticosteroid without regular monitoring.
- Try to minimise long-term topical corticosteroid use by introducing non-steroid preparations where possible. However, in lichen sclerosus, this is usually not feasible.
- Do not put pressure on patients to have breaks from treatment if this results in relapse.
- Always attempt to use ointments in preference to creams. These are better tolerated and less likely to cause irritation and allergy. Some patients hate ointments, and if they tolerate creams, then do not press the issue.
- Monitor for redness: this is a sign that you are using a topical corticosteroid that is too strong for your patient. Reduce to a lower strength, and the redness will then disappear over the next few weeks.
- Realise that 'thin skin' is very unlikely if you use topical corticosteroids in this way. It will be evidenced by tears during intercourse or striae. Both are usually seen only in unsupervised patients using potent preparations for long periods of time.

What to Do if a Medication Stings

There are several reasons that medications may cause stinging:

- It is inherent to the medication itself
- It is caused by a preservative or a product found in the base of a cream
- The patient's skin is very inflamed and fissured
- The patient has hyperalgesia associated with a neuropathy
- The patient has used too much potent topical corticosteroid so her skin is red and has become very sensitive

First, examine your patient for the presence of an underlying condition. If there is a severely inflamed dermatosis and no topical therapy is tolerated, it may be necessary to use a systemic agent long enough to control this before changing back to a topical agent.

In many cases, it will take a few days for the stinging to stop. If you suspect excess topical corticosteroid, reduce to a weaker preparation. If the examination is normal and you suspect hyperalgesia, stop all topical therapy.

If the patient is using a cream, cease this and change to an ointment. Certain topical therapies tend to sting even on intact skin, tacrolimus and pimecrolimus in particular. Some patients simply need an alternative product.

Tips to Optimise Compliance

Poor compliance tends to be related to:

- Fear of topical corticosteroids
- Cost of treatment
- The patient feeling well, and does not see the point of maintenance treatment
- The patient considering (perhaps falsely) her condition to be low risk
- Regimens that have to be applied multiple times per day
- Treatment regimens that recommend intermittent treatment; this often gets forgotten
- Treatment side effects
- Psychological barriers such as depression, denial or forgetfulness
- Embarrassment about having vaginal creams and pessaries where family members might find them
- Certain neuromodulators such as the tricyclic antidepressants, which still carry the stigma of being used for major depression

To optimise compliance:

- Make sure the patient understands the risks of non-compliance; in lichen sclerosus, this risk includes cancer and as a result, compliance is often excellent
- Ask your patient what she is worried about and what gets in the way and try to find solutions together
- Make sure the patient has the knowledge to know what is being treated and why
- Explain the concept of chronic disease and the difference between cure and control
- Give very strong reassurance about topical corticosteroids
- Explain that tricyclics are not being used as antidepressants
- Keep regimens simple, if possible once daily
- Minimise the cost of treatment to your patient in any way you can, by recommending economical products and by making them aware that they can shop around for the lowest price
- Make a follow-up visit appointment and remind your patient to attend

When to Refer a Patient to a Pelvic Floor Physiotherapist

The lower pelvic floor muscles lie directly under the skin of the vulva and vaginal mucosa. They frequently become hypertonic in response to vulvovaginal skin inflammation, leading to pain with stretch, and therefore to dyspareunia and pain with tampon insertion.

For most patients, this hypertonicity ('spasm') settles when the underlying cause improves. For others, it persists. Examination in this situation shows fixed spasm of the pubococcygeus muscle, with inability of the patient to either contract or relax the muscle. This persistent pelvic muscular spasm is often exacerbated by co-existing biomechanical problems, such as lumbosacral or hip joint dysfunction.

You should consider referral to a physiotherapist if:

- The patient's dyspareunia does not settle once the dermatosis is controlled
- There is evidence on examination of pubococcygeus spasm
- There is evidence of hyperalgesia

When to Refer a Patient to a Counsellor

Relative to the number of patients we encounter with vulval disease, we refer only a few to counsellors. It is not essential to refer every patient with a vulval problem for psychosexual help.

Many patients with straightforward skin diseases of the vulva recover quickly and resume normal sex lives without any assistance other than appropriate medical treatment.

The reasons we have referred in the past include:

- Relationship problems
- Sexual abuse
- Depression
- High levels of anger related to previous adverse experiences with the medical profession
- Obsessions with sexually transmissible infections
- Patients with pelvic floor spasm who do not have the confidence to resume intercourse after treatment
- Patients who are using their condition to manipulate others
- The very small group of patients with a genuinely psychosexual cause for their dyspareunia

When to Refer a Patient to a Pain Management Specialist

Patients with neuropathic vulval pain are often easily helped with neuromodulating medications, exercise, weight loss and physiotherapy.

However, there are those whose pain is intractable, has been present for many years and who have associated significant psychological problems. There is also a group where significant drug interactions with neuromodulators require a very expert prescriber.

Patients in this group need the expertise of a specialist in pain management. They frequently also need psychiatric help, although this suggestion tends to be less well received.

Should You Ever Tell a Patient You Have Nothing Further to Offer Her?

In the course of managing patients with vulval disease, we have often seen patients who claim that they have been told, sometimes on more than one occasion, that there is nothing that can be done to help them.

This possibly relates more to the very limited information that is available to doctors on the subject of vulval disease than to a limit on therapeutic options.

We certainly cannot help everyone. In some cases, we lack the skills. In some, psychological issues get in the way of effective compliance, making it difficult to ever achieve a good result from therapy.

If we feel that a patient's problems are beyond our area of expertise, we should leave them with a diagnosis and a referral to another practitioner whom we feel may be able to help. It is important to know when it is time for a patient to move on but not with a sense that 'there is nothing that anyone can do to help you'.

There is something that will help most patients, even if it is just a validation that their problem is real and deserves our serious attention. Nothing in medicine has been more neglected than the field of vulval disease.

Index